CONTENTS

INTRODUCTION

What is the Ninja Foodi 2-Basket Air Fryer?

The Ninja Foodi 2- Basket Air Fryer is the next revolutionary appliance coming from the awesome folks working at Ninja Kitchen! No matter how unbelievable the concept might sound, Ninja Kitchen has put on countless hours of engineering into crafting this meticulously designed appliance that takes the Air Frying game to a whole different level.

At its heart, the Ninja Foodi 2 Basket Air Fryer is a simple and exceedingly effective Air Fryer that gives you all the basic functions that you would expect from an Air Fryer. With this appliance, you can Air Frye, Bake, Broil, Dehydrate, Air Crisp, and more! You know, the usual Air Fryer stuffs.

However, what makes this unique is the super cool "Dual Zone" technology that completely flips the game in the Air Frying market.

If you are looking to cut down your cooking to half, or you want to make two different meals at the same time. The same appliance, then the Ninja Foodi Dual Zone/ 2 Basket Air Fryer is exactly what you need!

Simply put, the Dual Zone technology allows the appliance to be put on either single cook mode or multi cook mode.

Single cook mode works as usual; you cook using just a single basket. However, with the Dual Cook mode, you can seamlessly set the different timer, mode, and temperature for both of the zones individually and cook the meals you require.

Alternatively, you may give the same settings to both of the zones and cook the same meal in a doubled portion without spending any more time than you would need when making just a single portion.

While handling two Air Fryer baskets might sound a little bit complicated at first, the way how Ninja Kitchen has engineered this appliance has made it extremely accessible and easy to handle.

Understanding the functional buttons and features

The Dual Zone Air Fryer technology of this appliance has merged 6 different cooking functions such as Air Broil, Air Fry, Roast, Bake, Dehydrate and Reheat into one simple and easy to the appliance.

This appliance is extremely awesome for people who love the bake and cook crispy foods.

This particular Air Fryer comes with 2 different Fryer baskets, which are marked as 1 and 2. each should be inserted into their respective section of the appliance because of their different shapes.

Keep in mind that the baskets themselves don't have any buttons, so you can just pull them out and insert them as needed.

The display itself is divided into 2 different sections that indicate each section of the Basket settings. Pres Key -1 on the control panel to select Basket 1 setting and Key 2 for basket 2 settings.

Apart from that, the other functional buttons that you should know about include:

- **Air Broil:** This mode will allow you to give your meals a nice crispy finish and melt toppings of the food.
- **Air Fry:** This is the standard mode that you should use if you want to cook/fry food without using oil
- **Roast:** This essentially turns your appliance into a roaster oven that allows you to cook soft and tender meat
- **Bake:** This will allow you to bake awesome delicious desserts and treats
- **Reheat:** This will allow you to re-heat and warm your leftover meals
- **Dehydrate:** This feature will allow you to dehydrate meats, fruits, and vegetables.
- With the function buttons out of the way, the next thing you should focus on is the appliance's operating buttons.
- **Temp Key:** The Up and Down keys will allow you to adjust the cooking temperature.
- **Time Arrows:** The Up and Down keys here will allow you to adjust the cooking time.
- **SMART FINISH button:** This button will allow your appliance to automatically sync the times of both cooking zones and let them finish simultaneously.
- **MATCH COOK button:** This button will allow you to automatically match the settings of Zone 2 with that of Zone 1. This is amazing when you want to cook many cooks or a large portion of the same food.
- **START/PAUSE button:** These buttons will allow you to initiate, stop, and resume your meal's cooking.
- **POWER BUTTON:** This button is pressed to turn the appliance on and off when needed.
- **Hold Mode:** The Hold sign will appear on the display screen in the SMART FINISH mode. When the cooking time of one zone is greater than the other, the hold will appear for the zone with less cooking time as it will wait for the cooking of another zone to be complete.

Learning the functions work

To properly use the Ninja Foodi 2 Basket Air Fryer, you should have a good idea of the different cooking programs present in the appliance. While the previous section covered the different available functions, this section will tell you how to use them. We will go through them one by one.

Air Broil

- The first step is to insert the crisper plate in your cooking basket, add ingredients into the Basket and insert the Basket into the unit
- By default, the unit will use Zone 1; however, if you want to use zone 2, you need to select Zone 2
- Select the AIR BROIL cooking mode
- Use the TEMP keys to set the temperature that you need
- Use the TIME key to set your desired time
- Press the START/PAUSE button to start cooking
- Once the cooking is done, you will hear a beep, and an "End" sign will appear on the display
- Remove the cooked ingredients and serve

Air Fry

- The first step is to insert the crisper plate in your cooking basket, add ingredients into the Basket and insert the Basket into the unit
- By default, the unit will use Zone 1; however, if you want to use zone 2, you need to select Zone 2
- Select the AIR FRY cooking mode
- Use the TEMP keys to set the temperature that you need
- Use the TIME key to set your desired time
- Press the START/PAUSE button to start cooking
- Once the cooking is done, you will hear a beep, and an "End" sign will appear on the display
- Remove the cooked ingredients and serve

Bake

- The first step is to insert the crisper plate in your cooking basket, add ingredients into the Basket and insert the Basket into the unit
- Select the BAKE cooking mode
- Use the TEMP keys to set the temperature that you need
- Use the TIME key to set your desired time
- Press the START/PAUSE button to start cooking
- Once the cooking is done, you will hear a beep, and an "End" sign will appear on the display
- Keep in mind that you can reduce the temp by 25 degrees F while converting the traditional oven recipes for Air Fryer baking
- Remove the cooked ingredients and serve

For the other cooking modes available, the process is pretty simple. You will the same steps, select the crisper plate/cooking rack as needed, select the required mode, zone, and temperature then start cooking.

Keep in mind, though, that the broiling function is not available for the MATCH COOK technology, as the appliance only allows you to broil food in one Basket at a time. If you have many ingredients to broil, the best way is to broil in batches.

Thanks to the Dual-Zone technology, you have access to other exclusive features of the appliance.

MATCH COOK

If you want to cook a large amount of the same food, or you want to cook two different foods at the same time, here are the steps to follow:

- Add your cooking ingredients into the Basket, insert both baskets into the unit
- Zone 1 will stay lit; press your desired function button. Use the TEMP buttons to set the temperature, use the TIME key to set the desired time.
- Press the MATCH COOK button to copy the settings of basket 1 to that of basket 2
- Press the START/PAUSE button and initiate cooking in both baskets
- Once done, the "' End" sign will appear on both screens

SMART FINISH TECHNOLOGY

These functions will allow both of the cooking zones to complete their cooking simultaneously, even if both of the zones have completely different cook settings.

- Add listed ingredients to your Basket and then insert the baskets into the Air Fryer unit
- Press the Smart Finish Mode, and the machine will automatically sync during cooking
- At first, Zone 1 will stay illuminated. At this point, you need to choose the cooking function for this zone; use the TEMP key to fix temperature and TIME to set the time.
- Now select Zone 2, set the cooking function
- Use TEMP Keys to set temperature and Time key to set the cooking time for Zone 2.
- Once all is set, press the start button; the timer will start ticking for both of the zones according to the set timer, the cooking will finish simultaneously.
- On Smart Finish Mode, you can also start cooking simultaneously and let it end at different times. For that, simply select the cooking time and press the start button for both Zones

Hearty tips for using the appliance

Since this is a relatively new appliance to hit the market, people are still beginning to grasp this amazing appliance's full potential. They are exploring how to properly use this product. The following tips will greatly enhance your cooking experience with this appliance and make everything a breeze.

- While most of the required temperatures are already provided in the recipes, if you ever feel confused, just have a look at the cooking table provided in this book.
- It's always suggested that you collect all of the ingredients you require before starting your cooking session. If you are unable to find a specific ingredient, then make sure to find an alternative beforehand. The recipes in this book already have the best ingredients chosen to provide the best flavor. Still, since different people have different taste buds, you might consider altering a few if you feel like it.
- Make sure to read the recipes thoroughly before you start cooking; if you find any step confusing, then do a simple google search to properly understand the steps.
- Before starting your cooking session, make sure that your appliance to clean and free from any dirt or debris. Follow the steps provided in the section below if you are confused about how to do it.
- The Air Fryer location is extremely important if you want your meals to cook evenly since it relies heavily on the airflow. Therefore, make sure to keep it in a space where it has enough space to "Breath" in Air and cook the meals properly.
- If you are using frozen food, you should consider thawing them before putting them in your Air Fryer basket.
- Since the Air Fryer relies on Superheated Air to do the cooking, make sure to never overcrowd the cooking baskets. Always keep space in between heavy ingredients. Now that you have two zones to work with, this shouldn't be a problem at all!
- When cooking with the Air Fryer, it is always advised that you opt for organic ingredients. Try to find the freshest ones possible as they will give you the best flavors.

- When choosing a baking tray for your Air Fryer, try to go for lighter color trays/dishes. Dark colors such as black ones would absorb more heat that might result in uneven cooking.

Maintaining and cleaning the appliance

Despite having a bucket load of functions under its hood, cleaning up and maintain the Ninja Foodi 2 Basket Air Fryer is relatively easy. To clear up any confusion that you may have, let me break down the process into very simple and easy to follow steps.

- First of all, unplug the appliance before you start cleaning it, making sure that you have given it enough time to let it cool
- Next, remove the Air Fryer baskets from the main appliance and keep them on the side; this will help with the cooling process as well
- Once they are cool, remove the Air Crisper plates and wash them thoroughly
- Take the Air Fryer baskets and use soapy water to clean them; make sure to avoid using any hard scrubber as they might damage the surface
- The Air Fryer racks can be washed in Dishwasher; afterward, use a soft scrub to gently clean any food stuck to the sides
- Take the main unit, and gently wipe it using a clean piece of cloth
- Once everything is clean, return the Basket back to the Air Fryer
- And now, you are ready to go!

If you just follow these simple steps, you will be able to keep your 2 Basket Air Fryer in tip-top shape for days to come!

BREAKFAST & BRUNCH RECIPES

1. Sausages Casserole

Servings: 4

Cooking Time: 25 Minutes

Ingredients:

- 3 spring onions, chopped
- 1 green bell pepper, sliced
- ¼ teaspoon salt
- ¼ teaspoon ground turmeric
- ¼ teaspoon ground paprika
- 10 oz Italian sausages
- 1 teaspoon olive oil
- 4 eggs

Directions:

1. Preheat the air fryer to 360F. Then pour olive oil in the air fryer basket. Add bell pepper and spring onions. Then sprinkle the vegetables with ground turmeric and salt. Cook them for 5 minutes. When the time is finished, shake the air fryer basket gently. Chop the sausages roughly and add in the air fryer basket. Cook the ingredients for 10 minutes. Then crack the eggs over the sausages and cook the casserole for 10 minutes more.

2. Scallion Wontons

Servings: 4

Cooking Time: 2 Minutes

Ingredients:

- ½ teaspoon garlic powder
- 1 oz scallions, chopped
- 1 teaspoon fresh dill, chopped
- 4 tablespoons cream cheese
- 8 wonton wraps
- Cooking spray

Directions:

1. In the mixing bowl mix up garlic powder, scallions, fresh dill, and cream cheese. Then fill the wonton wraps with cream cheese mixture and fold them. Preheat the air fryer to 355F. Place the wonton wraps in the air fryer basket and cook them for 2 minutes or until they are light brown.

3. Apple Bran Granola

Servings: 4

Cooking Time: 15 Minutes

Ingredients:

- ½ cup granola
- ½ cup bran flakes
- 2 green apples, cored, peeled and roughly chopped
- ¼ cup apple juice
- ⅛ cup maple syrup
- 2 tablespoons butter
- 1 teaspoon cinnamon powder

Directions:

1. In your air fryer, mix all ingredients.
2. Toss, cover, and cook at 365 degrees F for 15 minutes.
3. Divide into bowls and serve; enjoy!

4. Breakfast Banana Bread

Servings:2

Cooking Time: 50 Minutes

Ingredients:

- 1 tbsp flour
- ¼ tsp baking soda
- 1 tsp baking powder
- ⅓ cup sugar
- 2 mashed bananas
- ¼ cup vegetable oil
- 1 egg, beaten
- 1 tsp vanilla extract
- ¾ cup chopped walnuts

- ¼ tsp salt
- 2 tbsp peanut butter
- 2 tbsp sour cream
- Cooking spray

Directions:

1. Preheat the air fryer to 330 F. Spray a small baking dish, that fits inside, with cooking spray or grease with butter. Combine the flour, salt, baking powder, and baking soda, in a bowl.
2. In another bowl, combine bananas, oil, egg, peanut butter, vanilla, sugar, and sour cream. Mix both mixtures. Stir in chopped walnuts. Pour the batter into the dish. Cook for 40 minutes and serve chill.

5. Delicious Doughnuts

Servings: 6
Cooking Time:28 Minutes
Ingredients:

- 1/2 cup sugar
- 1/3 cup caster sugar
- 4 tbsp. butter; soft
- 1 ½ tsp. baking powder
- 2 an 1/4 cups white flour
- 1 tsp. cinnamon powder
- 2 egg yolks
- 1/2 cup sour cream

Directions:

1. In a bowl; mix 2 tbsp. butter with simple sugar and egg yolks and whisk well.
2. Add half of the sour cream and stir.
3. In another bowls; mix flour with baking powder, stir and also add to eggs mix.
4. Stir well until you obtain a dough, transfer it to a floured working surface; roll it out and cut big circles with smaller ones in the middle.

5. Brush doughnuts with the rest of the butter; heat up your air fryer at 360 degrees F; place doughnuts inside and cook them for 8 minutes.
6. In a bowl; mix cinnamon with caster sugar and stir. Arrange doughnuts on plates and dip them in cinnamon and sugar before serving.

6. Green Beans And Eggs

Servings: 4
Cooking Time: 20 Minutes
Ingredients:

- 1 pound green beans, roughly chopped
- Cooking spray
- 2 eggs, whisked
- Salt and black pepper to the taste
- 1 tablespoon sweet paprika
- 4 ounces sour cream

Directions:

1. Grease a pan that fits your air fryer with the cooking spray and mix all the ingredients inside. Put the pan in the Air Fryer and cook at 360 degrees F for 20 minutes. Divide between plates and serve.

7. Chives Yogurt Eggs

Servings: 4
Cooking Time: 20 Minutes
Ingredients:

- Cooking spray
- Salt and black pepper to the taste
- 1 and ½ cups Greek yogurt
- 4 eggs, whisked
- 1 tablespoon chives, chopped
- 1 tablespoon cilantro, chopped

Directions:

1. In a bowl, mix all the ingredients except the cooking spray and whisk well. Grease a pan that fits the air

fryer with the cooking spray, pour the eggs mix, spread well, put the pan into the machine and cook the omelet at 360 degrees F for 20 minutes. Divide between plates and serve for breakfast.

8. Bacon And Egg Bite Cups

Servings:4
Cooking Time:15 Minutes
Ingredients:
- 6 large eggs
- ½ cup red peppers, chopped
- ¼ cup fresh spinach, chopped
- ¾ cup mozzarella cheese, shredded
- 3 slices bacon, cooked and crumbled
- 2 tablespoons heavy whipping cream
- Salt and black pepper, to taste

Directions:
1. Preheat the Air fryer to 300 °F and grease 4 silicone molds.
2. Whisk together eggs with cream, salt and black pepper in a large bowl until combined.
3. Stir in rest of the ingredients and transfer the mixture into silicone molds.
4. Place in the Air fryer and cook for about 15 minutes.
5. Dish out and serve warm.

9. Great Japanese Omelette

Servings:1
Cooking Time: 20 Minutes
Ingredients:
- 3 whole eggs
- Black pepper to taste
- 1 tsp coriander
- 1 tsp cumin
- 2 tbsp soy sauce
- 2 tbsp green onion, chopped
- Olive oil

- 1 whole onion, chopped

Directions:
1. In a bowl, mix eggs, soy sauce, cumin, pepper, oil, and salt. Add cubed tofu to baking forms and pour the egg mixture on top. Place the prepared forms in the air fryer cooking basket and cook for 10 minutes at 400 F. Serve with a sprinkle of coriander and green onion.

10. Breakfast Muffins

Servings: 1
Cooking Time: 30 Minutes
Ingredients:
- 1 medium egg
- ¼ cup heavy cream
- 1 slice cooked bacon (cured, pan-fried, cooked)
- 1 oz cheddar cheese
- Salt and black pepper (to taste)

Directions:
1. Preheat your fryer to 350°F/175°C.
2. In a bowl, mix the eggs with the cream, salt and pepper.
3. Spread into muffin tins and fill the cups half full.
4. Place 1 slice of bacon into each muffin hole and half ounce of cheese on top of each muffin.
5. Bake for around 15-20 minutes or until slightly browned.
6. Add another ½ oz of cheese onto each muffin and broil until the cheese is slightly browned. Serve!

11. Cheesy Omelet

Servings:1
Cooking Time: 15 Minutes
Ingredients:
- Black pepper to taste
- 1 cup cheddar cheese, shredded

- 1 whole onion, chopped
- 2 tbsp soy sauce

Directions:
1. Preheat your air fryer to 340 F. Drizzle soy sauce over the chopped onions. Place the onions in your air fryer's cooking basket and cook for 8 minutes. In a bowl, mix the beaten eggs with salt and pepper.
2. Pour the egg mixture over onions (in the cooking basket) and cook for 3 minutes. Add cheddar cheese over eggs and bake for 2 more minutes. Serve with fresh basil and enjoy!

12. Broccoli Frittata

Servings: 2
Cooking Time: 17 Minutes
Ingredients:
- 3 eggs
- 1/2 cup bell pepper, chopped
- 1/2 cup broccoli florets
- 2 tbsp parmesan cheese, grated
- 1/4 tsp garlic powder
- 1/4 tsp onion powder
- 2 tbsp coconut milk
- Pepper
- Salt

Directions:
1. Spray air fryer baking dish with cooking spray.
2. Place bell peppers and broccoli in the prepared baking dish.
3. Cook broccoli and bell pepper in the air fryer at 350 F for 7 minutes.
4. In a bowl, whisk together eggs, milk, and seasoning.
5. Once veggies are cooked then pour egg mixture over vegetables and sprinkle cheese on top.

6. Cook frittata in the air fryer for 10 minutes.
7. Serve and enjoy.

13. Special Shrimp Sandwiches

Servings: 4
Cooking Time:15 Minutes
Ingredients:
- 1 ¼ cups cheddar; shredded
- 2 tbsp. green onions; chopped.
- 4 whole wheat bread slices
- 6 oz. canned tiny shrimp; drained
- 3 tbsp. mayonnaise
- 2 tbsp. butter; soft

Directions:
1. In a bowl; mix shrimp with cheese, green onion and mayo and stir well.
2. Spread this on half of the bread slices; top with the other bread slices, cut into halves diagonally and spread butter on top.
3. Place sandwiches in your air fryer and cook at 350 °F, for 5 minutes. Divide shrimp sandwiches on plates and serve them for breakfast.

14. Vegetable Toast

Servings: 4
Cooking Time: 25 Minutes
Ingredients:
- 4 slices bread
- 1 red bell pepper, cut into strips
- 1 cup sliced button or cremini mushrooms
- 1 small yellow squash, sliced
- 2 green onions, sliced
- 1 tbsp. olive oil
- 2 tbsp. softened butter
- ½ cup soft goat cheese

Directions:
1. Drizzle the Air Fryer with the olive oil and pre-heat to 350°F.

2. Put the red pepper, green onions, mushrooms, and squash inside the fryer, give them a stir and cook for 7 minutes, shaking the basket once throughout the cooking time. Ensure the vegetables become tender.
3. Remove the vegetables and set them aside.
4. Spread some butter on the slices of bread and transfer to the Air Fryer, butter side-up. Brown for 2 to 4 minutes.
5. Remove the toast from the fryer and top with goat cheese and vegetables. Serve warm.

15. Coffee Donuts

Servings: 6
Cooking Time: 20 Minutes
Ingredients:
- 1 cup flour
- ¼ cup sugar
- ½ tsp. salt
- 1 tsp. baking powder
- 1 tbsp. aquafaba
- 1 tbsp. sunflower oil
- ¼ cup coffee

Directions:
1. In a large bowl, combine the sugar, salt, flour, and baking powder.
2. Add in the coffee, aquafaba, and sunflower oil and mix until a dough is formed. Leave the dough to rest in and the refrigerator.
3. Set your Air Fryer at 400°F to heat up.
4. Remove the dough from the fridge and divide up, kneading each section into a doughnut.
5. Put the doughnuts inside the Air Fryer, ensuring not to overlap any. Fry for 6 minutes. Do not shake the

basket, to make sure the doughnuts hold their shape.

16. Apple Muffins

Servings:12
Cooking Time: 25 Minutes
Ingredients:
- 1¾ cups plain flour
- 1/3 cup white sugar
- 1½ teaspoons baking powder
- ½ teaspoon ground cinnamon
- ¼ teaspoon ground ginger
- ¼ teaspoon salt
- ¾ cup milk
- 1/3 cup applesauce
- 1 cup apple, cored and chopped

Directions:
1. In a large bowl, mix together the flour, sugar, baking powder, spices, and salt.
2. Add in the milk and applesauce. Beat until just combined.
3. Fold in the chopped apple.
4. Set the temperature of Air Fryer to 390 degrees F. Grease 12 muffin molds.
5. Put the mixture evenly into the prepared muffin molds.
6. Arrange the molds into an Air Fryer basket.
7. Air Fry for about 20-25 minutes or until a toothpick inserted in the center comes out clean.
8. Remove the muffin molds from Air Fryer and place onto a wire rack to cool for about 10 minutes.
9. Carefully, invert the muffins onto the wire rack to completely cool before serving.
10. Serve.

17. Cheddar Hash Browns

Servings:4

Cooking Time: 25 Minutes

Ingredients:

- 1 brown onion, chopped
- 3 garlic cloves, chopped
- ½ cup grated cheddar cheese
- 1 egg, lightly beaten
- Salt and black pepper
- 3 tbsp finely thyme sprigs
- Cooking spray

Directions:

1. In a bowl, mix with hands potatoes, onion, garlic, cheese, egg, salt, black pepper, and thyme. Spray the fryer with cooking spray.
2. Press the hash brown mixture into the basket and cook for 9 minutes at 400 F., shaking once halfway through cooking. When ready, ensure the hash browns are golden and crispy.

18. Air Fried Calzone

Servings:4

Cooking Time: 20 Minutes

Ingredients:

- 4 oz cheddar cheese, grated
- 1 oz mozzarella cheese
- 1 oz bacon, diced
- 2 cups cooked and shredded turkey
- 1 egg, beaten
- 4 tbsp tomato paste
- 1 tsp basil
- 1 tsp oregano
- Salt and pepper, to taste

Directions:

1. Preheat the air fryer to 350 F. Divide the pizza dough into 4 equal pieces so you have the dough for 4 small pizza crusts. Combine the tomato paste, basil, and oregano in a small bowl.
2. Brush the mixture onto the crusts, just make sure not to go all the way

and avoid brushing near the edges on one half of each crust, place ½ turkey, and season the meat with some salt and pepper. Top the meat with bacon. Divide mozzarella and cheddar cheeses between pizzas. Brush the edges with beaten egg. Fold the crust and seal with a fork. Cook for 10 minutes.

19. Blueberry Muffins

Servings:12

Cooking Time: 12 Minutes

Ingredients:

- 2 cups plus 2 tablespoons self-rising flour
- 5 tablespoons white sugar
- ½ cup milk
- 2 ounces butter, melted
- 2 eggs
- 2 teaspoons fresh orange zest, finely grated
- 2 tablespoons fresh orange juice
- ½ teaspoon vanilla extract
- ½ cup fresh blueberries

Directions:

1. In a bowl, mix together the flour, and white sugar.
2. In another large bowl, mix well the remaining ingredients except blueberries.
3. Now, add in the flour mixture and mix until just combined.
4. Fold in the blueberries.
5. Set the temperature of Air Fryer to 355 degrees F. Grease 12 muffin molds.
6. Put the mixture evenly into the prepared muffin molds. Arrange the molds into an Air Fryer basket.

7. Air Fry for about 12 minutes or until a toothpick inserted in the center comes out clean.
8. Remove the muffin molds from Air Fryer and place onto a wire rack to cool for about 10 minutes.
9. Carefully, invert the muffins onto the wire rack to completely cool before serving.
10. Serve.

20. Air Fryer Breakfast Casserole

Servings:2
Cooking Time:25 Minutes
Ingredients:
- 3 red potatoes
- 3 eggs
- 2 turkey sausage patties
- ¼ cup cheddar cheese
- 1 tablespoon milk
- Olive oil cooking spray

Directions:
1. Preheat the Air fryer to 400 ° F and grease a baking dish with cooking spray.
2. Place the potatoes in the Air fryer basket and cook for about 10 minutes.
3. Whisk eggs with milk in a bowl.
4. Put the potatoes and sausage in the baking dish and pour egg mixture on top.
5. Sprinkle with cheddar cheese and arrange in the Air fryer.
6. Cook for about 15 minutes at 350 ° F and dish out to serve warm.

21. Tomato And Greens Salad

Servings: 4
Cooking Time: 15 Minutes
Ingredients:
- 1 teaspoon olive oil
- 2 cups mustard greens

- A pinch of salt and black pepper
- ½ pound cherry tomatoes, cubed
- 2 tablespoons chives, chopped

Directions:
1. Heat up your air fryer with the oil at 360 degrees F, add all the ingredients, toss, cook for 15 minutes shaking halfway, divide into bowls and serve for breakfast.

22. Sweet Potato Hash

Servings:6
Cooking Time:15 Minutes
Ingredients:
- 2 large sweet potato, cut into small cubes
- 2 slices bacon, cut into small pieces
- 2 tablespoons olive oil
- 1 tablespoon smoked paprika
- 1 teaspoon sea salt
- 1 teaspoon ground black pepper
- 1 teaspoon dried dill weed

Directions:
1. Preheat the Air Fryer to 400 °F and grease an Air fryer pan.
2. Mix together sweet potato, bacon, olive oil, paprika, salt, black pepper and dill in a large bowl.
3. Transfer the mixture into the preheated air fryer pan and cook for about 15 minutes, stirring in between.
4. Dish out and serve warm.

23. Egg Muffins

Servings: 1
Cooking Time: 30 Minutes
Ingredients:
- 1 tbsp green pesto
- oz/75g shredded cheese
- oz/150g cooked bacon
- 1 scallion, chopped

- eggs

Directions:

1. You should set your fryer to 350°F/175°C.
2. Place liners in a regular cupcake tin. This will help with easy removal and storage.
3. Beat the eggs with pepper, salt, and the pesto. Mix in the cheese.
4. Pour the eggs into the cupcake tin and top with the bacon and scallion.
5. Cook for 15-20 minutes, or until the egg is set.

24. Sausage Quiche

Servings: 4
Cooking Time: 35 Minutes
Ingredients:

- 12 large eggs
- 1 cup heavy cream
- 1 tsp black pepper
- 12 oz sugar-free breakfast sausage
- 2 cups shredded cheddar cheese

Directions:

1. Preheat your fryer to 375°F/190°C.
2. In a large bowl, whisk the eggs, heavy cream, salad and pepper together.
3. Add the breakfast sausage and cheddar cheese.
4. Pour the mixture into a greased casserole dish.
5. Bake for 25 minutes.
6. Cut into 12 squares and serve hot.

25. Three Meat Cheesy Omelet

Servings:2
Cooking Time: 20 Minutes
Ingredients:

- 4 slices prosciutto, chopped
- 3 oz salami, chopped
- 1 cup grated mozzarella cheese
- 4 eggs

- 1 tbsp chopped onion
- 1 tbsp ketchup

Directions:

1. Preheat the air fryer to 350 F. Whisk eggs with ketchup in a bowl. Stir in onion. Cook the sausage in the air fryer for 2 minutes. Combine the egg mixture, mozzarella cheese, salami and prosciutto. Pour the egg mixture over the sausage and stir. Cook for 10 minutes.

26. Chicken Muffins

Servings: 6
Cooking Time: 10 Minutes
Ingredients:

- 1 cup ground chicken
- 1 cup ground pork
- ½ cup Mozzarella, shredded
- 1 teaspoon dried oregano
- ½ teaspoon salt
- 1 teaspoon ground paprika
- ½ teaspoon white pepper
- 1 tablespoon ghee, melted
- 1 teaspoon dried dill
- 2 tablespoons almond flour
- 1 egg, beaten

Directions:

1. In the bowl mix up ground chicken, ground pork, dried oregano, salt, ground paprika, white pepper, dried dill, almond flour, and egg. When you get the homogenous texture of the mass, add ½ of all Mozzarella and mix up the mixture gently with the help of the spoon. Then brush the silicone muffin molds with melted ghee. Put the meat mixture in the muffin molds. Flatten the surface of every muffin with the help of the spoon and top with remaining Mozzarella. Preheat

the air fryer to 375F. Then arrange the muffins in the air fryer basket and cook them for 10 minutes. Cool the cooked muffins to the room temperature and remove from the muffin molds.

27. Broccoli Casserole

Servings: 4
Cooking Time: 25 Minutes
Ingredients:
- 1 broccoli head, florets separated and roughly chopped
- 2 ounces cheddar cheese, grated
- 4 eggs, whisked
- 1 cup almond milk
- 2 teaspoons cilantro, chopped
- Salt and black pepper to the taste

Directions:
1. In a bowl, mix the eggs with the milk, cilantro, salt and pepper and whisk. Put the broccoli in your air fryer, add the eggs mix over it, spread, sprinkle the cheese on top, cook at 350 degrees F for 25 minutes, divide between plates and serve for breakfast.

28. Mozzarella Rolls

Servings: 6
Cooking Time: 6 Minutes
Ingredients:
- 6 wonton wrappers
- 1 tablespoon keto tomato sauce
- ½ cup Mozzarella, shredded
- 1 oz pepperoni, chopped
- 1 egg, beaten
- Cooking spray

Directions:
1. In the big bowl mix up together shredded Mozzarella, pepperoni, and tomato sauce. When the mixture is

homogenous transfer it on the wonton wraps. Wrap the wonton wraps in the shape of sticks. Then brush them with beaten eggs. Preheat the air fryer to 400F. Spray the air fryer basket with cooking spray. Put the pizza sticks in the air fryer and cook them for 3 minutes from each side.

29. Buttered Eggs In Hole

Servings:2
Cooking Time: 11 Minutes
Ingredients:
- 2 eggs
- Salt and pepper to taste
- 2 tbsp butter

Directions:
1. Place a heatproof bowl in the fryer's basket and brush with butter. Make a hole in the middle of the bread slices with a bread knife and place in the heatproof bowl in 2 batches. Break an egg into the center of each hole. Season with salt and pepper. Close the air fryer and cook for 4 minutes at 330 F. Turn the bread with a spatula and cook for another 4 minutes. Serve as a breakfast accompaniment.

30. Taj Tofu

Servings: 4
Cooking Time: 40 Minutes
Ingredients:
- 1 block firm tofu, pressed and cut into 1-inch thick cubes
- 2 tbsp. soy sauce
- 2 tsp. sesame seeds, toasted
- 1 tsp. rice vinegar
- 1 tbsp. cornstarch

Directions:
1. Set your Air Fryer at 400°F to warm.

2. Add the tofu, soy sauce, sesame seeds and rice vinegar in a bowl together and mix well to coat the tofu cubes. Then cover the tofu in cornstarch and put it in the basket of your fryer.
3. Cook for 25 minutes, giving the basket a shake at five-minute intervals to ensure the tofu cooks evenly.

31. Black's Bangin' Casserole

Servings: 4
Cooking Time: 40 Minutes
Ingredients:
- 5 eggs
- 3 tbsp chunky tomato sauce
- 2 tbsp heavy cream
- 2 tbsp grated parmesan cheese

Directions:
1. Preheat your fryer to 350°F/175°C.
2. Combine the eggs and cream in a bowl.
3. Mix in the tomato sauce and add the cheese.
4. Spread into a glass baking dish and bake for 25-35 minutes.
5. Top with extra cheese.
6. Enjoy!

LUNCH & DINNER RECIPES

32. Pesto Stuffed Bella Mushrooms

Servings: 6
Cooking Time: 25 Minutes
Ingredients:

- 1 cup basil
- ½ cup cashew nuts, soaked overnight
- ½ cup nutritional yeast
- 1 tbsp. lemon juice
- 2 cloves of garlic
- 1 tbsp. olive oil
- Salt to taste
- 1 lb. baby Bella mushroom, stems removed

Directions:

1. Pre-heat the Air Fryer at 400°F.
2. Prepare your pesto. In a food processor, blend together the basil, cashew nuts, nutritional yeast, lemon juice, garlic and olive oil to combine well. Sprinkle on salt as desired.
3. Turn the mushrooms cap-side down and spread the pesto on the underside of each cap.
4. Transfer to the fryer and cook for 15 minutes.

33. Chicken Lunch Recipe

Servings: 6
Cooking Time:30 Minutes
Ingredients:

- 1 bunch kale; chopped
- 1 cup chicken; shredded
- 3 carrots; chopped
- 1 cup shiitake mushrooms; roughly sliced
- 1/4 cup chicken stock
- Salt and black pepper to the taste

Directions:

1. In a blender, mix stock with kale, pulse a few times and pour into a pan that fits your air fryer. Add chicken, mushrooms, carrots, salt and pepper to the taste; toss, introduce in your air fryer and cook at 350 °F, for 18 minutes.

34. Zucchini Casserole

Servings: 4
Cooking Time: 30 Minutes
Ingredients:

- 1 cup ground chicken
- ½ cup ground pork
- 2 oz celery stalk, chopped
- 1 zucchini, grated
- 1 tablespoon coconut oil, melted
- ½ teaspoon salt
- 1 teaspoon ground black pepper
- ½ teaspoon chili flakes
- 1 teaspoon dried dill
- ½ teaspoon dried parsley
- ½ cup beef broth

Directions:

1. In the mixing bowl mix up ground chicken, ground pork, celery stalk, and salt. Add ground black pepper, chili flakes, dried dill, and dried parsley. Stir the meat mixture until homogenous. Then brush the air fryer pan with coconut oil and put ½ part of all grated zucchini. Then spread it with all ground pork mixture. Sprinkle the meat with remaining grated zucchini and cover with foil. Preheat the air fryer to 375F. Place the pan with casserole in the air fryer and cook it for 25 minutes. When the time is finished, remove the foil and

cook the casserole for 5 minutes more.

35. Sweet & Sour Tofu

Servings: 2
Cooking Time: 55 Minutes
Ingredients:
- 2 tsp. apple cider vinegar
- 1 tbsp. sugar
- 1 tbsp. soy sauce
- 3 tsp. lime juice
- 1 tsp. ground ginger
- 1 tsp. garlic powder
- ½ block firm tofu, pressed to remove excess liquid and cut into cubes
- 1 tsp. cornstarch
- 2 green onions, chopped
- Toasted sesame seeds for garnish

Directions:
1. In a bowl, thoroughly combine the apple cider vinegar, sugar, soy sauce, lime juice, ground ginger, and garlic powder.
2. Cover the tofu with this mixture and leave to marinate for at least 30 minutes.
3. Transfer the tofu to the Air Fryer, keeping any excess marinade for the sauce. Cook at 400°F for 20 minutes or until crispy.
4. In the meantime, thicken the sauce with the cornstarch over a medium-low heat.
5. Serve the cooked tofu with the sauce, green onions, sesame seeds, and some rice.

36. Chicken Corn Casserole

Servings: 6
Cooking Time:40 Minutes
Ingredients:
- 1 cup clean chicken stock
- 6 oz. canned coconut milk
- 1 ½ cups green lentils
- 2 lbs. chicken breasts; skinless, boneless and cubed
- 1/3 cup cilantro; chopped
- 3 cups corn
- 3 handfuls spinach
- 3 green onions; chopped
- 2 tsp. garlic powder
- Salt and black pepper to the taste

Directions:
1. In a pan that fits your air fryer; mix stock with coconut milk, salt, pepper, garlic powder, chicken and lentils. Add corn, green onions, cilantro and spinach; stir well, introduce in your air fryer and cook at 350 °F, for 30 minutes.

37. Lamb Stew

Servings: 4
Cooking Time: 30 Minutes
Ingredients:
- 1 cup eggplant, cubed
- 2 garlic cloves, minced
- 3 celery ribs, chopped
- ½ cups keto tomato sauce
- 1 pound lamb stew meat, cubed
- 1 tablespoon olive oil
- Salt and black pepper to the taste

Directions:
1. Heat up a pan that fits the air fryer with the oil over medium-high heat, add the lamb, salt, pepper and the garlic and brown for 5 minutes. Add the rest of the ingredients, toss, introduce the pan in the machine and cook at 370 degrees F for 25 minutes. Divide into bowls and serve for lunch.

38. Portabella Pizza

Servings: 3
Cooking Time: 15 Minutes
Ingredients:

- 3 tbsp. olive oil
- 3 portobello mushroom caps, cleaned and scooped
- 3 tbsp. mozzarella, shredded
- 3 tbsp. tomato sauce
- Pinch of salt
- 12 slices pepperoni
- Pinch of dried Italian seasonings

Directions:

1. Pre-heat the Air Fryer to 330°F.
2. Coat both sides of the mushroom cap with a drizzle of oil, before seasoning the inside with the Italian seasonings and salt. Evenly spread the tomato sauce over the mushroom and add the cheese on top.
3. Put the mushroom into the cooking basket of the Air Fryer. Place the slices of pepperoni on top of the portobello pizza after a minute of cooking and continue to cook for another 3-5 minutes.

39. Rosemary Rib Eye Steaks

Servings: 2
Cooking Time: 40 Minutes
Ingredients:

- ¼ cup butter
- 1 clove minced garlic
- Salt and pepper
- 1 ½ tbsp. balsamic vinegar
- ¼ cup rosemary, chopped
- 2 ribeye steaks

Directions:

1. Melt the butter in a skillet over medium heat. Add the garlic and fry until fragrant.
2. Remove the skillet from the heat and add in the salt, pepper, and vinegar. Allow it to cool.
3. Add the rosemary, then pour the whole mixture into a Ziploc bag.
4. Put the ribeye steaks in the bag and shake well, making sure to coat the meat well. Refrigerate for an hour, then allow to sit for a further twenty minutes.
5. Pre-heat the fryer at 400°F and set the rack inside. Cook the ribeyes for fifteen minutes.
6. Take care when removing the steaks from the fryer and plate up. Enjoy!

40. Italian Lamb Chops

Servings: 2
Cooking Time: 20 Minutes
Ingredients:

- 2 lamp chops
- 2 tsp. Italian herbs
- 2 avocados
- ½ cup mayonnaise
- 1 tbsp. lemon juice

Directions:

1. Season the lamb chops with the Italian herbs, then set aside for five minutes.
2. Pre-heat the fryer at 400°F and place the rack inside.
3. Put the chops on the rack and allow to cook for twelve minutes.
4. In the meantime, halve the avocados and open to remove the pits. Spoon the flesh into a blender.
5. Add in the mayonnaise and lemon juice and pulse until a smooth consistency is achieved.
6. Take care when removing the chops from the fryer, then plate up and serve with the avocado mayo.

41. Chili Beef Bowl

Servings: 3
Cooking Time: 18 Minutes
Ingredients:

- 9 oz beef sirloin
- 1 chili pepper
- 1 green bell pepper
- ½ teaspoon minced garlic
- ¼ teaspoon ground ginger
- 1 tablespoon apple cider vinegar
- 4 tablespoons water
- ½ teaspoon salt
- 3 spring onions, chopped
- 1 teaspoon avocado oil

Directions:

1. Cut the beef sirloin into wedges. Then cut bell pepper and chili pepper into wedges. Put bell pepper, chili pepper, and beef sirloin in the bowl. Add minced garlic, ground ginger, apple cider vinegar, water, salt, and spring onions. Marinate the mixture for 15 minutes. Meanwhile, preheat the air fryer to 210F. Put the bell pepper, chili pepper, and onion in the air fryer basket. Sprinkle them with ½ teaspoon of avocado oil and cook them for 8 minutes. Transfer the cooked vegetables in 3 serving bowls. After this, put the beef wedges in the air fryer and sprinkle them with remaining avocado oil. Cook the meat for 10 minutes at 365F. Stir it from time to time to avoid burning. Meanwhile, pour the marinade from the beef and vegetables in the saucepan and bring it to boil. Simmer it for 2-3 minutes. Put the cooked beef in the serving bowls. Sprinkle the meal with hot marinade.

42. Creamy Zucchini Noodle Mix

Servings: 2
Cooking Time: 9 Minutes
Ingredients:

- 1 zucchini, trimmed
- 4 oz chicken breast, skinless, boneless
- ¼ cup heavy cream
- 2 oz Parmesan, grated
- ½ teaspoon ground black pepper
- ¼ teaspoon ground paprika
- ½ teaspoon sesame oil
- ½ teaspoon dried basil

Directions:

1. Make the zoodles from the zucchini with the help of the spiralizer. Then rub the chicken breast with ground black pepper, paprika, and basil. Sprinkle the chicken breast with sesame oil and put it in the air fryer. Cook it for 8 minutes at 400F. Flip the chicken on another side after 4 minutes of cooking. When the chicken is cooked, remove it from the air fryer and place it on the plate. Then put the zucchini zoodles in the air fryer and cook then at 400F for 1 minute. Meanwhile, mix up parmesan and heavy cream and preheat the liquid over the medium heat until the cheese is melted. Then mix up heavy cream sauce and zucchini. Mix it up well. Chop the chicken roughly and top the zoodles with it.

43. Bacon Pancetta Casserole

Servings: 4
Cooking Time: 20 Minutes
Ingredients:

- 2 cups cauliflower, shredded
- 3 oz pancetta, chopped

- 2 oz bacon, chopped
- 1 cup Cheddar cheese, shredded
- ½ cup heavy cream
- 1 teaspoon salt
- 1 teaspoon cayenne pepper
- 1 teaspoon dried oregano

Directions:
1. Put bacon and pancetta in the air fryer and cook it for 10 minutes at 400F. Stir the ingredients every 3 minutes to avoid burning. Then mix up shredded cauliflower and cooked pancetta and bacon. Add salt and cayenne pepper. Mix up the mixture. Add the dried oregano. Line the air fryer pan with baking paper and put the cauliflower mixture inside. Top it with Cheddar cheese and sprinkle with heavy cream. Cook the casserole for 10 minutes at 365F.

44. Beef Chili

Servings: 4
Cooking Time: 29 Minutes
Ingredients:
- 2 spring onions, chopped
- 2 medium green bell peppers, chopped
- 1 tablespoon avocado oil
- ½ teaspoon salt
- ½ teaspoon ground black pepper
- 2 cups ground beef
- 1 teaspoon ground paprika
- 1 teaspoon chili flakes
- ½ teaspoon white pepper
- 1 teaspoon ground cumin
- ½ teaspoon ground coriander
- 1 chili pepper, chopped
- 1 cup beef broth
- 1 tablespoon keto tomato sauce
- 1 cup lettuce leaves

Directions:
1. Put the spring onions in the air fryer pan. Add green bell peppers, avocado oil, salt, and ground black pepper. Stir the mixture gently. Preheat the air fryer to 365F and place the pan with vegetables inside. Cook them for 4 minutes. Then stir well. In the mixing bowl mix up ground beef, ground paprika, chili flakes, white pepper, ground cumin, ground coriander, and tomato sauce Put the meat mixture over the vegetables and carefully stir it with the help of the spoon. Add chili pepper and beef broth. Stir the chili gently. Cook it at 365F for 25 minutes. Stir the chili every 5 minutes of cooking. When the chili is cooked, cool it for 5-10 minutes. Then fill the lettuce leaves with chili and transfer in the serving plates.

45. Cashew & Chicken Manchurian

Servings: 6
Cooking Time: 30 Minutes
Ingredients:
- 1 cup chicken boneless
- 1 spring onions, chopped
- 1 onion, chopped
- 3 green chili
- 6 cashew nuts
- 1 tsp. ginger, chopped
- ½ tsp. garlic, chopped
- 1 Egg
- 2 tbsp. flour
- 1 tbsp. cornstarch
- 1 tsp. soy sauce
- 2 tsp. chili paste
- 1 tsp. pepper
- Pinch MSG
- sugar as needed

- 1 tbsp. oil

Directions:

1. Pre-heat your Air Fryer at 360°F
2. Toss together the chicken, egg, salt and pepper to coat well.
3. Combine the cornstarch and flour and use this to cover the chicken.
4. Cook in the fryer for 10 minutes.
5. In the meantime, toast the nuts in a frying pan. Add in the onions and cook until they turn translucent. Combine with the remaining ingredients to create the sauce.
6. Finally, add in the chicken. When piping hot, garnish with the spring onions and serve.

46. Chicken Rolls

Servings: 4
Cooking Time: 18 Minutes

Ingredients:

- 2 large zucchini
- ½ cup Cheddar cheese, shredded
- 1-pound chicken breast, skinless, boneless
- 1 teaspoon dried oregano
- ½ teaspoon olive oil
- 1 teaspoon salt
- 2 spring onions, chopped
- 1 teaspoon ground paprika
- ½ teaspoon ground turmeric
- ½ cup keto tomato sauce

Directions:

1. Preheat the skillet well and pour the olive oil inside. Put the onions in it and sprinkle with salt, ground paprika, and ground turmeric. Cook the onion for 5 minutes over the medium-high heat. Stir it from time to time. Meanwhile, shred the chicken. Add it in the skillet. Then add oregano. Stir well and cook the mixture for 2 minutes. After this, remove the skillet from the heat. Cut the zucchini into halves (lengthwise). Then make the zucchini slices with the help of the vegetable peeler. Put 3 zucchini slices on the chopping board overlapping each of them. Then spread the surface of them with the shredded chicken mixture. Roll the zucchini carefully in the shape of the roll. Repeat the same steps with remaining zucchini and shredded chicken mixture. Line the air fryer pan with parchment and put the enchilada rolls inside. Sprinkle them with tomato sauce Preheat the air fryer to 350F. Top the zucchini rolls (enchiladas) with Cheddar cheese and put in the air fryer basket. Cook the meal for 10 minutes.

47. Cabbage Stew

Servings: 4
Cooking Time: 20 Minutes

Ingredients:

- 14 ounces tomatoes, chopped
- 1 green cabbage head, shredded
- Salt and black pepper to the taste
- 1 tablespoon sweet paprika
- 4 ounces chicken stock
- 2 tablespoon dill, chopped

Directions:

1. In a pan that fits your air fryer, mix the cabbage with the tomatoes and all the other ingredients except the dill, toss, introduce the pan in the fryer, and cook at 380 degrees F for 20 minutes. Divide into bowls and serve with dill sprinkled on top.

48. Pork Casserole

Servings: 6
Cooking Time: 30 Minutes
Ingredients:

- 1 teaspoon taco seasonings
- 1 teaspoon sesame oil
- 1 teaspoon salt
- 2 cups ground pork
- ½ cup keto tomato sauce
- 2 low carb tortillas
- ½ cup Cheddar cheese, shredded
- ¼ cup mozzarella cheese, shredded

Directions:

1. Chop the tortillas roughly. Brush the air fryer pan with sesame oil and place ½ part of chopped tortilla in it. In the mixing bowl mix up taco seasonings, ground pork, and salt. Place ½ part of ground pork over the tortillas and top it with mozzarella cheese. Then cover the cheese with remaining tortillas, ground pork, and Cheddar cheese. Pour the marinara sauce over the cheese and cover the casserole with foil. Secure the edges. Preheat the air fryer to 395F. Put the casserole in the air fryer and cook it for 20 minutes. Then remove the foil and cook it for 10 minutes more.

49. Lunch Baby Carrots Mix

Servings: 4
Cooking Time: 15 Minutes
Ingredients:

- 16 ounces baby carrots
- Salt and black pepper to taste
- 2 tablespoons butter, melted
- 4 ounces chicken stock
- 2 tablespoons dill, chopped

Directions:

1. In a pan that fits your air fryer, mix all the ingredients and toss.
2. Place the pan in the fryer and cook at 380 degrees F for 15 minutes.
3. Divide between bowls and serve.

50. Chicken And Asparagus

Servings: 4
Cooking Time: 20 Minutes
Ingredients:

- 4 chicken breasts, skinless, boneless and halved
- 1 tablespoon sweet paprika
- 1 bunch asparagus, trimmed and halved
- 1 tablespoon olive oil
- Salt and black pepper to the taste

Directions:

1. In a bowl, mix all the ingredients, toss, put them in your Air Fryer's basket and cook at 390 degrees F for 20 minutes. Divide between plates and serve for lunch.

51. Radish And Tuna Salad

Servings: 2
Cooking Time: 8 Minutes
Ingredients:

- ½ cup radish sprouts
- 8 oz tuna, smoked, boneless and shredded
- 1 egg, beaten
- 1 tablespoon coconut flour
- ½ teaspoon ground coriander
- ½ teaspoon lemon zest, grated
- 1 tablespoon olive oil
- ½ teaspoon salt
- 1 tablespoon lemon juice
- ½ cup radish, sliced

Directions:

1. Mix up the tuna with coconut flour, ground coriander, lemon zest, and egg. Stir the mixture until homogenous. Preheat the air fryer to 400F. Then make the small tuna balls and put them in the hot air fryer. Sprinkle the tuna balls with ½ tablespoon of olive oil. Cook the tuna balls for 8 minutes. Flip the tuna balls on another side after 4 minutes of cooking. Meanwhile, mix up together radish sprouts and radish. Sprinkle the mixture with remaining olive oil, salt, and lemon juice. Shake it well. Then top the salad with tuna balls.

52. Fiery Jalapeno Poppers

Servings: 4
Cooking Time: 40 Minutes
Ingredients:
- 5 oz cream cheese
- ¼ cup mozzarella cheese
- 8 medium jalapeno peppers
- ½ tsp Mrs. Dash Table Blend
- 8 slices bacon

Directions:
1. Preheat your fryer to 400°F/200°C.
2. Cut the jalapenos in half.
3. Use a spoon to scrape out the insides of the peppers.
4. In a bowl, add together the cream cheese, mozzarella cheese and spices of your choice.
5. Pack the cream cheese mixture into the jalapenos and place the peppers on top.
6. Wrap each pepper in 1 slice of bacon, starting from the bottom and working up.
7. Bake for 30 minutes. Broil for an additional 3 minutes.
8. Serve!

53. Oregano Cod And Arugula Mix

Servings: 4
Cooking Time: 12 Minutes
Ingredients:
- 2 tablespoons fresh cilantro, minced
- 1 pound cod fillets, boneless, skinless and cubed
- 1 spring onion, chopped
- Salt and black pepper to the taste
- ½ teaspoon sweet paprika
- ½ teaspoon oregano, ground
- A drizzle of olive oil
- 2 cups baby arugula

Directions:
1. In a bowl, mix the cod with salt, pepper, paprika, oregano and the oil, toss, transfer the cubes to your air fryer's basket and cook at 360 degrees F for 12 minutes. In a salad bowl, mix the cod with the remaining ingredients, toss, divide between plates and serve.

54. Lemon Dill Trout

Servings: 1
Cooking Time: 10 Minutes
Ingredients:
- 2 lb pan-dressed trout (or other small fish), fresh or frozen
- 1 ½ tsp salt
- ½ cup butter or margarine
- 2 tbsp dill weed
- 3 tbsp lemon juice

Directions:
1. Cut the fish lengthwise and season the with pepper.
2. Prepare a skillet by melting the butter and dill weed.
3. Fry the fish on a high heat, flesh side down, for 2-3 minutes per side.

4. Remove the fish. Add the lemon juice to the butter and dill to create a sauce.
5. Serve the fish with the sauce.

55. Chili Sloppy Joes

Servings: 3
Cooking Time: 20 Minutes
Ingredients:
- 1 cup ground pork
- 1 teaspoon sloppy Joes seasonings
- 1 teaspoon butter
- 1 tablespoon keto tomato sauce
- 1 teaspoon mustard
- ¼ cup beef broth
- ½ teaspoon chili flakes
- ½ bell pepper, chopped
- ½ teaspoon minced garlic

Directions:
1. In the bowl mix up chili flakes, beef broth, minced garlic, and tomato sauce. Add mustard and whisk the liquid until homogenous. After this, add ground pork and sloppy Joes seasonings. Stir the ingredients with the help of the spoon and transfer in the air fryer baking pan. Add butter. Preheat the air fryer to 365F. Put the pan with sloppy Joe in the air fryer basket and cook the meal for 20 minutes. Stir the meal well after 10 minutes of cooking.

56. Spiced Beef Meatballs

Servings: 2
Cooking Time: 10 Minutes
Ingredients:
- 1 oz pimiento jalapenos, pickled, chopped
- ½ teaspoon dried rosemary
- ½ teaspoon salt
- 9 oz ground beef
- ½ teaspoon ground coriander
- ¼ teaspoon ground nutmeg
- 1 egg, beaten
- 2 oz provolone cheese, shredded
- 2 teaspoons mascarpone
- ¼ teaspoon minced garlic
- Cooking spray

Directions:
1. In the mixing bowl mix up pickled pimiento jalapenos, dried rosemary, salt, ground beef, coriander, nutmeg, egg, and make the medium-size meatballs. Preheat the air fryer to 365F. Then spray the air fryer basket with cooking spray and place the meatballs inside. Cook the meatballs for 6 minutes, Then carefully flip them on another side and cook for 4 minutes more. Meanwhile, churn together minced garlic and mascarpone. When the meatballs are cooked, transfer them in the serving plates and top with garlic mascarpone.

57. Cayenne Zucchini Mix

Servings: 2
Cooking Time: 16 Minutes
Ingredients:
- 2 zucchini
- ½ cup Monterey jack cheese, shredded
- ¼ cup ground chicken
- 1 teaspoon salt
- ½ teaspoon cayenne pepper
- 1 teaspoon olive oil

Directions:
1. Trim the zucchini and cut it into the Hasselback. In the mixing bowl mix up ground chicken, cheese, salt, and cayenne pepper. The fill the zucchini with chicken mixture and sprinkle

with olive oil. Preheat the air fryer to 400F. Put the Hasselback zucchini in the air fryer and cook for 16 minutes at 400F.

58. Masala Meatloaf

Servings: 4
Cooking Time: 20 Minutes
Ingredients:
- 2 cups ground beef
- 1 large egg, beaten
- 2 spring onions, chopped
- 1teaspoon garam masala
- ½ teaspoon ground ginger
- 1 teaspoon garlic powder
- ½ teaspoon salt
- ½ teaspoon ground turmeric
- ½ teaspoon cayenne pepper
- 1 teaspoon olive oil
- ¼ teaspoon ground nutmeg

Directions:
1. In the mixing bowl mix up ground beef, egg, onion, garam masala, ground ginger, garlic powder, salt, ground turmeric, cayenne pepper, and ground nutmeg. Stir the mass with the help of the spoon until homogenous. Then brush the round air fryer pan with olive oil and place the ground beef mixture inside. Press the meatloaf gently. Place the pan with meatloaf in the air fryer and cook for 20 minutes at 365F.

59. Salsa Chicken Mix

Servings: 4
Cooking Time: 17 Minutes
Ingredients:
- 4 chicken breasts, skinless, boneless and cubed
- 2 tablespoons olive oil
- 1 onion, chopped

- 3 garlic cloves, minced
- 16 ounces jarred chunky salsa
- 20 ounces canned tomatoes, peeled and chopped
- Salt and black pepper to taste
- 2 tablespoons parsley, dried
- 1 teaspoon garlic powder
- 1 tablespoon chili powder
- 12 ounces canned black beans, drained

Directions:
1. Place all ingredients into a pan that fits your air fryer and toss.
2. Put the pan in the fryer and cook at 380 degrees F for 17 minutes.
3. Divide into bowls, serve, and enjoy.

60. Cheddar Bacon Burst

Servings: 8
Cooking Time: 90 Minutes
Ingredients:
- 30 slices bacon
- 2 ½ cups cheddar cheese
- 4-5 cups raw spinach
- 1-2 tbsp Tones Southwest Chipotle Seasoning
- 2 tsp Mrs. Dash Table Seasoning

Directions:
1. Preheat your fryer to 375°F/190°C.
2. Weave the bacon into 15 vertical pieces & 12 horizontal pieces. Cut the extra 3 in half to fill in the rest, horizontally.
3. Season the bacon.
4. Add the cheese to the bacon.
5. Add the spinach and press down to compress.
6. Tightly roll up the woven bacon.
7. Line a baking sheet with kitchen foil and add plenty of salt to it.

8. Put the bacon on top of a cooling rack and put that on top of your baking sheet.
9. Bake for 60-70 minutes.
10. Let cool for 10-15 minutes before
11. Slice and enjoy!

61. Flank Steak & Avocado Butter

Servings: 1
Cooking Time: 40 Minutes
Ingredients:
- 1 flank steak
- Salt and pepper
- 2 avocados
- 2 tbsp. butter, melted
- ½ cup chimichurri sauce

Directions:
1. Rub the flank steak with salt and pepper to taste and leave to sit for twenty minutes.
2. Pre-heat the fryer at 400°F and place a rack inside.
3. Halve the avocados and take out the pits. Spoon the flesh into a bowl and mash with a fork. Mix in the melted butter and chimichurri sauce, making sure everything is well combined.
4. Put the steak in the fryer and cook for six minutes. Flip over and allow to cook for another six minutes.
5. Serve the steak with the avocado butter and enjoy!

62. Parmesan Chicken

Servings: 4
Cooking Time: 30 Minutes
Ingredients:
- 1 teaspoon olive oil
- 4 spring onions, chopped
- 2 chicken breasts, skinless, boneless and cubed
- Salt and black pepper to the taste
- 1 and ½ cups parmesan cheese, grated
- ½ cup keto tomato sauce

Directions:
1. Preheat your air fryer at 400 degrees F, add half of the oil and the spring onions and fry them for 8 minutes, shaking the fryer halfway. Add the rest of the ingredients, toss, cook at 370 degrees F for 22 minutes, shaking the fryer halfway as well. Divide between plates and serve for lunch.

VEGETABLE & SIDE DISHES

63. Potato Gratin

Servings: 6
Cooking Time: 55 Minutes
Ingredients:

- ½ cup milk
- 7 medium russet potatoes, peeled
- 1 tsp. black pepper
- ½ cup cream
- ½ cup semi-mature cheese, grated
- ½ tsp. nutmeg

Directions:

1. Pre-heat the Air Fryer to 390°F.
2. Cut the potatoes into wafer-thin slices.
3. In a bowl, combine the milk and cream and sprinkle with salt, pepper, and nutmeg as desired.
4. Use the milk mixture to coat the slices of potatoes. Place in an 8" heat-resistant baking dish. Top the potatoes with the rest of the cream mixture.
5. Put the baking dish into the basket of the fryer and cook for 25 minutes.
6. Pour the cheese over the potatoes.
7. Cook for an additional 10 minutes, ensuring the top is nicely browned before serving.

64. Easy Sesame Broccoli

Servings: 3
Cooking Time: 15 Minutes
Ingredients:

- 1 pound broccoli florets
- 2 tablespoons sesame oil
- 1/2 teaspoon shallot powder
- 1/2 teaspoon porcini powder
- 1 teaspoon garlic powder
- Sea salt and ground black pepper, to taste
- 1/2 teaspoon cumin powder
- 1/4 teaspoon paprika
- 2 tablespoons sesame seeds

Directions:

1. Start by preheating the Air Fryer to 400 degrees F.
2. Blanch the broccoli in salted boiling water until al dente, about 3 to 4 minutes. Drain well and transfer to the lightly greased Air Fryer basket.
3. Add the sesame oil, shallot powder, porcini powder, garlic powder, salt, black pepper, cumin powder, paprika, and sesame seeds.
4. Cook for 6 minutes, tossing halfway through the cooking time. Bon appétit!

65. Garlic Tomatoes Recipe

Servings: 4
Cooking Time:25 Minutes
Ingredients:

- 4 garlic cloves; crushed
- 1 lb. mixed cherry tomatoes
- 3 thyme springs; chopped.
- 1/4 cup olive oil
- Salt and black pepper to the taste

Directions:

1. In a bowl; mix tomatoes with salt, black pepper, garlic, olive oil and thyme, toss to coat, introduce in your air fryer and cook at 360 °F, for 15 minutes. Divide tomatoes mix on plates and serve

66. Garlic Fried Mushrooms

Servings: 4
Cooking Time: 15 Minutes
Ingredients:

- 1 pound button mushrooms
- 1 ½ cups pork rinds
- 1 cup parmesan cheese, grated
- 2 eggs, whisked
- 1/2 teaspoon salt
- 2 tablespoons fresh parsley leaves, roughly chopped

Directions:
1. Pat the mushrooms dry with a paper towel.
2. To begin, set up your "breading" station. Mix the pork rinds and parmesan cheese in a shallow dish. In a separate dish, whisk the eggs.
3. Start by dipping the mushrooms into the eggs. Press your mushrooms into the parm/pork rind mixture, coating evenly.
4. Spritz the Air Fryer basket with cooking oil. Add the mushrooms and cook at 400 degrees F for 6 minutes, flipping them halfway through the cooking time.
5. Sprinkle with the salt. Serve garnished with fresh parsley leaves. Bon appétit!

67. Coconut Parmesan Kale

Servings: 4
Cooking Time: 15 Minutes
Ingredients:
- 2 pounds kale, torn
- A pinch of salt and black pepper
- 2 tablespoons olive oil
- 2 garlic cloves, minced
- 1 and ½ cups coconut cream
- ½ teaspoon nutmeg, ground
- ½ cup parmesan, grated

Directions:
1. In a pan that fits your air fryer, mix the kale with the rest of the

ingredients, toss, introduce the pan in the fryer and cook at 400 degrees F for 15 minutes. Divide between plates and serve.

68. Roasted Brussels Sprout Salad

Servings: 2
Cooking Time: 35 Minutes + Chilling Time
Ingredients:
- 1/2 pound Brussels sprouts
- 1 tablespoon olive oil
- Coarse sea salt and ground black pepper, to taste
- 2 ounces baby arugula
- 1 shallot, thinly sliced
- 2 ounces pancetta, chopped
- Lemon Vinaigrette:
- 2 tablespoons extra virgin olive oil
- 2 tablespoons fresh lemon juice
- 1 tablespoon honey
- 1 teaspoon Dijon mustard

Directions:
1. Start by preheating your Air Fryer to 380 degrees F.
2. Add the Brussels sprouts to the cooking basket. Brush with olive oil and cook for 15 minutes. Let it cool to room temperature about 15 minutes.
3. Toss the Brussels sprouts with the salt, black pepper, baby arugula, and shallot.
4. Mix all ingredients for the dressing. Then, dress your salad, garnish with pancetta, and serve well chilled. Bon appétit!

69. Fried Creamy Cabbage

Servings: 4
Cooking Time:30 Minutes
Ingredients:
- 1 green cabbage head; chopped.
- 1 yellow onion; chopped.

- 4 bacon slices; chopped.
- 1 cup whipped cream
- 2 tbsp. cornstarch
- Salt and black pepper to the taste

Directions:

1. Put cabbage, bacon and onion in your air fryer.
2. In a bowl; mix cornstarch with cream, salt and pepper, stir and add over cabbage. Toss, cook at 400 °F, for 20 minutes; divide among plates and serve as a side dish.

70. Yellow Squash And Zucchinis Dish

Servings: 4
Cooking Time:45 Minutes
Ingredients:

- 1 yellow squash; halved, deseeded and cut into chunks
- 6 tsp. olive oil
- 1 lb. zucchinis; sliced
- 1/2 lb. carrots; cubed
- 1 tbsp. tarragon; chopped
- Salt and white pepper to the taste

Directions:

1. In your air fryer's basket; mix zucchinis with carrots, squash, salt, pepper and oil; toss well and cook at 400 °F, for 25 minutes. Divide them on plates and serve as a side dish with tarragon sprinkled on top.

71. Simple Taro Fries

Servings: 2
Cooking Time: 20 Minutes
Ingredients:

- 8 small taro, peel and cut into fries shape
- 1 tbsp olive oil
- 1/2 tsp salt

Directions:

1. Add taro slice in a bowl and toss well with olive oil and salt.
2. Transfer taro slices into the air fryer basket.
3. Cook at 360 F for 20 minutes. Toss halfway through.
4. Serve and enjoy.

72. Rainbow Vegetable Fritters

Servings: 2
Cooking Time: 20 Minutes
Ingredients:

- 1 zucchini, grated and squeezed
- 1 cup corn kernels
- 1/2 cup canned green peas
- 4 tablespoons all-purpose flour
- 2 tablespoons fresh shallots, minced
- 1 teaspoon fresh garlic, minced
- 1 tablespoon peanut oil
- Sea salt and ground black pepper, to taste
- 1 teaspoon cayenne pepper

Directions:

1. In a mixing bowl, thoroughly combine all ingredients until everything is well incorporated.
2. Shape the mixture into patties. Spritz the Air Fryer basket with cooking spray.
3. Cook in the preheated Air Fryer at 365 degrees F for 6 minutes. Turn them over and cook for a further 6 minutes
4. Serve immediately and enjoy!

73. Pesto Pasta

Servings: 4
Cooking Time: 15 Minutes
Ingredients:

- 2 cups zucchinis, cut with a spiralizer
- Salt and black pepper to the taste
- 1 tablespoon olive oil

- ½ cup coconut cream
- 4 ounces mozzarella, shredded
- ¼ cup basil pesto

Directions:

1. In a pan that fits your air fryer, mix the zucchini noodles with the pesto and the rest of the ingredients, toss, introduce the pan in the fryer and cook at 370 degrees F for 15 minutes. Divide between plates and serve as a side dish.

74. Lime Olives And Zucchini

Servings: 4
Cooking Time: 12 Minutes
Ingredients:

- 4 zucchinis, sliced
- 1 cup kalamata olives, pitted
- Salt and black pepper to the taste
- 2 tablespoons lime juice
- 2 tablespoons olive oil
- 2 teaspoons balsamic vinegar

Directions:

1. In a pan that fits your air fryer, mix the olives with all the other ingredients, toss, introduce in the fryer and cook at 390 degrees F for 12 minutes. Divide the mix between plates and serve.

75. Dilled Asparagus With Cheese

Servings: 3
Cooking Time: 15 Minutes
Ingredients:

- 1 bunch of asparagus, trimmed
- 1 tablespoon olive oil
- 1/2 teaspoon kosher salt
- 1/4 teaspoon cracked black pepper, to taste
- 1/2 teaspoon dried dill weed
- 1/2 cup goat cheese, crumbled

Directions:

1. Place the asparagus spears in the lightly greased cooking basket. Toss the asparagus with the olive oil, salt, black pepper, and dill.
2. Cook in the preheated Air Fryer at 400 degrees F for 9 minutes.
3. Serve garnished with goat cheese. Bon appétit!

76. Chives Endives

Servings: 4
Cooking Time: 15 Minutes
Ingredients:

- 4 endives, trimmed
- A pinch of salt and black pepper
- ¼ cup goat cheese, crumbled
- 1 teaspoon lemon zest, grated
- 1 tablespoon lemon juice
- 2 tablespoons chives, chopped
- 2 tablespoons olive oil

Directions:

1. In a bowl, mix the endives with the other ingredients except the cheese and chives and toss well. Put the endives in your air fryer's basket and cook at 380 degrees F for 15 minutes. Divide the corn between plates and serve with cheese and chives sprinkled on top.

77. Easy Shepherd's Pie

Servings: 5
Cooking Time: 30 Minutes
Ingredients:

- 2 tablespoons olive oil
- 2 bell peppers, seeded and sliced
- 1 celery, chopped
- 1 onion, chopped
- 2 garlic cloves, minced
- 1 cup cooked bacon, diced
- 1 ½ cups beef bone broth

- 5 ounces green beans, drained
- Sea salt and freshly ground black pepper, to taste
- 8 ounces cauliflower pulsed in a food processor to a fine-crumb like consistency
- 1/2 cup milk
- 2 tablespoons butter, melted

Directions:

1. Heat the olive oil in a saucepan over medium-high heat. Now, cook the peppers, celery, onion, and garlic until they have softened, about 7 minutes
2. Add the bacon and broth. Bring to a boil and cook for 2 minutes more. Stir in green beans, salt and black pepper; continue to cook until everything is heated through.
3. Transfer the mixture to the lightly greased baking pan.
4. Microwave cauliflower rice for 5 minutes.
5. In a small bowl, combine the cauliflower, milk, and melted butter. Stir until well mixed and spoon evenly over the vegetable mixture. Smooth it with a spatula and transfer to the Air Fryer cooking basket.
6. Bake in the preheated Air Fryer at 400 degrees F for 12 minutes. Place on a wire rack to cool slightly before slicing and serving. Bon appétit!

78. Simple Cauliflower Bars

Servings: 12
Cooking Time:35 Minutes
Ingredients:

- 1 big cauliflower head; florets separated
- 1 tsp. Italian seasoning

- 1/2 cup mozzarella; shredded
- 1/4 cup egg whites
- Salt and black pepper to the taste

Directions:

1. Put cauliflower florets in your food processor; pulse well, spread on a lined baking sheet that fits your air fryer, introduce in the fryer and cook at 360 °F, for 10 minutes.
2. Transfer cauliflower to a bowl; add salt, pepper, cheese, egg whites and Italian seasoning; stir really well, spread this into a rectangle pan that fits your air fryer; press well, introduce in the fryer and cook at 360 °F, for 15 minutes more. Cut into 12 bars, arrange them on a platter and serve as a snack

79. Italian-style Broccoli

Servings: 4
Cooking Time: 25 Minutes
Ingredients:

- 1/3 cup Asiago cheese
- 1 large-sized head broccoli, stemmed and cut small florets
- 2 1/2 tablespoons canola oil
- 1 tablespoon Italian seasoning blend
- Salt and ground black pepper, to taste

Directions:

1. Bring a medium pan filled with a lightly salted water to a boil. Then, boil the broccoli florets for about 3 minutes.
2. Then, drain the broccoli florets well; toss them with the canola oil, rosemary, basil, salt and black pepper.
3. Set your Air Fryer to 390 degrees F; arrange the seasoned broccoli in the cooking basket; set the timer for 17

minutes. Toss the broccoli halfway through the cooking process.

4. Serve warm topped with grated cheese and enjoy!

80. Veggie Rolls

Servings: 6
Cooking Time: 30 Minutes
Ingredients:

- 2 potatoes, mashed
- ¼ cup peas
- ¼ cup carrots, mashed
- 1 small cabbage, sliced
- ¼ beans
- 2 tbsp. sweetcorn
- 1 small onion, chopped
- 1 tsp. capsicum
- 1 tsp. coriander
- 2 tbsp. butter
- Ginger
- Garlic to taste
- ½ tsp. masala powder
- ½ tsp. chili powder
- ½ cup bread crumbs
- 1 packet spring roll sheets
- ½ cup cornstarch slurry

Directions:

1. Boil all the vegetables in water over a low heat. Rinse and allow to dry.
2. Unroll the spring roll sheets and spoon equal amounts of vegetable onto the center of each one. Fold into spring rolls and coat each one with the slurry and bread crumbs.
3. Pre-heat the Air Fryer to 390°F. Cook the rolls for 10 minutes.
4. Serve with a side of boiled rice.

81. Swiss Asparagus

Servings: 4
Cooking Time: 6 Minutes

Ingredients:

- 12 oz asparagus, trimmed
- 2 eggs, beaten
- ¼ cup Swiss cheese, shredded
- ½ cup coconut flour
- 1 teaspoon olive oil
- 1 teaspoon salt

Directions:

1. In the mixing bowl mix up Swiss cheese, coconut flour, and salt. Then dip the asparagus in the beaten eggs and coat in the coconut flour mixture. Repeat the same steps one more time and transfer the coated asparagus in the air fryer basket. Cook the vegetables for 6 minutes at 395F.

82. Prosciutto & Cheese Stromboli

Servings:4
Cooking Time: 35 Minutes
Ingredients:

- 4 slices fontina cheese
- ½ cup shredded mozzarella cheese
- 8 slices prosciutto
- 16 halved cherry tomatoes
- 4 fresh basil leaves, chopped
- ½ tsp oregano
- Salt and black pepper to taste

Directions:

1. On lightly floured work surface, roll the pizza crust out. Slice in 4 squares. Top each piece with a slice of fontina cheese, 2 slices of prosciutto, 4 halved cherry tomatoes, oregano, and basil. Season with salt and pepper. Close the rectangle by folding in half, press and seal the edges with a fork. Spritz with cooking spray and transfer to air fryer. Cook for 15 minutes, turning once. Let cool to serve.

83. Collard Greens Sauté

Servings: 4
Cooking Time: 12 Minutes
Ingredients:
- 1 pound collard greens, trimmed
- 2 fennel bulbs, trimmed and quartered
- 2 tablespoons olive oil
- Salt and black pepper to the taste
- ½ cup keto tomato sauce

Directions:
1. In a pan that fits your air fryer, mix the collard greens with the fennel and the rest of the ingredients, toss, put the pan in the fryer and cook at 350 degrees F for 12 minutes. Divide everything between plates and serve.

84. Okra Salad

Servings: 2
Cooking Time: 6 Minutes
Ingredients:
- 6 oz okra, sliced
- 3 oz green beans, chopped
- 1 cup arugula, chopped
- 1 teaspoon lemon juice
- 1 teaspoon olive oil
- ½ teaspoon salt
- 2 eggs, beaten
- 1 tablespoon coconut flakes
- Cooking spray

Directions:
1. In the mixing bowl mix up sliced okra and green beans. Add cooking spray and salt and mix up the mixture well. Then add beaten eggs and shake it. After this, sprinkle the vegetables with coconut flakes and shake okra and green beans to coat them in the coconut flakes. Preheat the air fryer to 400F. Put the vegetable mixture in the air fryer and cook it for 6 minutes. Shake the mixture after 3 minutes of cooking. After this, mix up cooked vegetables with arugula, lemon juice, and sprinkle with olive oil. Shake the salad.

85. Thyme Mushroom Pan

Servings: 2
Cooking Time: 8 Minutes
Ingredients:
- 1/2 pound cremini mushrooms, sliced
- 1 cup coconut cream
- 1 teaspoon avocado oil
- ¼ teaspoon minced garlic
- ½ teaspoon dried thyme

Directions:
1. In the air fryer's pan, mix the mushrooms with the cream and the other ingredients, toss and cook at 380 degrees F for 8 minutes. Divide into bowls and serve.

86. Artichokes Sauté

Servings: 4
Cooking Time: 15 Minutes
Ingredients:
- 10 ounces artichoke hearts, halved
- 3 garlic cloves
- 2 cups baby spinach
- ¼ cup veggie stock
- 2 teaspoons lime juice
- Salt and black pepper to the taste

Directions:
1. In a pan that fits your air fryer, mix all the ingredients, toss, introduce in the fryer and cook at 370 degrees F for 15 minutes. Divide between plates and serve as a side dish.

87. Roasted Cauliflower & Broccoli

Servings: 6
Cooking Time: 15 Minutes
Ingredients:

- 3 cups cauliflower florets
- 3 cups broccoli florets
- 1/4 tsp paprika
- 1/2 tsp garlic powder
- 2 tbsp olive oil
- 1/8 tsp pepper
- 1/4 tsp sea salt

Directions:

1. Preheat the air fryer to 400 F.
2. Add broccoli in microwave-safe bowl and microwave for 3 minutes. Drain well.
3. Add broccoli in a large mixing bowl. Add remaining ingredients and toss well.
4. Transfer broccoli and cauliflower mixture into the air fryer basket and cook for 12 minutes.
5. Toss halfway through.
6. Serve and enjoy.

88. Crusted Coconut Shrimp

Servings:5
Cooking Time: 30 Minutes
Ingredients:

- ¾ cup shredded coconut
- 1 tbsp maple syrup
- ½ cup breadcrumbs
- ⅓ cup cornstarch
- ½ cup milk

Directions:

1. Pour the cornstarch and shrimp in a zipper bag and shake vigorously to coat. Mix the syrup and milk in a bowl and set aside. In a separate bowl, mix the breadcrumbs and shredded coconut. Open the zipper bag and remove shrimp while shaking off excess starch.
2. Dip shrimp in the milk mixture and then in the crumb mixture. Place in the fryer. Cook 12 minutes at 350 F, flipping once halfway through. Cook until golden brown. Serve with a coconut-based dip.

89. Bacon Cabbage

Servings: 2
Cooking Time: 12 Minutes
Ingredients:

- 8 oz Chinese cabbage, roughly chopped
- 2 oz bacon, chopped
- 1 tablespoon sunflower oil
- ½ teaspoon onion powder
- ½ teaspoon salt

Directions:

1. Cook the bacon at 400F for 10 minutes. Stir it from time to time. Then sprinkle it with onion powder and salt. Add Chinese cabbage and shake the mixture well. Cook it for 2 minutes. Then add sunflower oil, stir the meal and place in the serving plates.

90. Cheesy Omelet With Mixed Greens

Servings: 2
Cooking Time: 17 Minutes
Ingredients:

- 1/3 cup Ricotta cheese
- 5 eggs, beaten
- 1/2 red bell pepper, seeded and sliced
- 1 cup mixed greens, roughly chopped
- 1/2 green bell pepper, seeded and sliced
- 1/2 teaspoon dried basil
- 1/2 chipotle pepper, finely minced

- 1/2 teaspoon dried oregano

Directions:
1. Lightly coat the inside of a baking dish with a pan spray.
2. Then, throw all ingredients into the baking dish; give it a good stir.
3. Bake at 325 degrees F for 15 minutes.

91. Dill Tomato

Servings: 2
Cooking Time: 8 Minutes
Ingredients:
- 1 oz Parmesan, sliced
- 1 tomato
- 1 teaspoon fresh dill, chopped
- 1 teaspoon olive oil
- ¼ teaspoon dried thyme

Directions:
1. Trim the tomato and slice it on 2 pieces. Then preheat the air fryer to 350F. Top the tomato slices with sliced Parmesan, chopped fresh dill, and thyme. Sprinkle the tomatoes with olive oil and put in the air fryer. Cook the meal for 8 minutes. Remove cooked tomato parm from the air fryer with the help of the spatula.

92. Air Fried Vegetable Tempura

Servings:3
Cooking Time: 20 Minutes
Ingredients:
- 1 cup broccoli florets
- 1 red bell pepper, cut into strips
- 1 small sweet potato, peeled and cut into thick slices
- 1 small zucchini, cut into thick slices
- ⅔ cup cornstarch
- ⅓ cup all-purpose flour

- 1 egg, beaten
- ¾ cup club soda
- 1½ cups panko breadcrumbs
- Non-stick cooking spray

Directions:
1. Mix the cornstarch and all-purpose flour. Dredge the vegetables in this mixture.
2. Mix egg and club soda. Dip each flour-coated vegetable into this mixture soda before dredging in bread crumbs.
3. Place the vegetables on the double layer rack accessory and spray with cooking oil.
4. Place inside the air fryer.
5. Close and cook for 20 minutes at 350 °F.

93. Herby Meatballs

Servings:4
Cooking Time: 30 Minutes
Ingredients:
- 1 onion, finely chopped
- 3 garlic cloves, finely chopped
- 2 eggs
- 1 cup breadcrumbs
- ½ cup fresh mixed herbs
- Salt and pepper to taste
- Olive oil

Directions:
1. In a bowl, add beef, onion, garlic, eggs, crumbs, herbs, salt and pepper and mix with hands to combine. Shape into balls and arrange them in the air fryer's basket. Drizzle with oil and cook for 16 minutes at 380 F, turning once halfway through.

VEGAN & VEGETARIAN RECIPES

94. Mushrooms With Peas

Servings:4
Cooking Time:15 Minutes
Ingredients:

- 16 ounces cremini mushrooms, halved
- ½ cup frozen peas
- ½ cup soy sauce
- 4 tablespoons maple syrup
- 4 tablespoons rice vinegar
- 4 garlic cloves, finely chopped
- 2 teaspoons Chinese five spice powder
- ½ teaspoon ground ginger

Directions:

1. Preheat the Air fryer to 350 °F and grease an Air fryer pan.
2. Mix soy sauce, maple syrup, vinegar, garlic, five spice powder, and ground ginger in a bowl.
3. Arrange the mushrooms in the Air fryer basket and cook for about 10 minutes.
4. Stir in the soy sauce mixture and peas and cook for about 5 more minutes.
5. Dish out the mushroom mixture in plates and serve hot.

95. Baked Mediterranean Veggies

Servings:8
Cooking Time: 10 Minutes
Ingredients:

- 18 oz eggplant, cubed
- 4 garlic cloves, minced
- 18 oz zucchini, sliced
- A bunch of thyme sprig
- 18 oz bell pepper, sliced and deseeded
- Salt and pepper to taste
- 4 whole onions, chopped
- 18 oz tomatoes, sliced
- Breadcrumb as needed

Directions:

1. Preheat air fryer to 380 F. In a bowl, mix eggplant, garlic, oil, spices, and transfer the mix to the cooking basket; cook for 4 minutes. Add zucchini, tomatoes, bell pepper, onion, and bake for 6 minutes. Serve.

96. Sweet And Spicy Parsnips

Servings:6
Cooking Time:44 Minutes
Ingredients:

- 2 pounds parsnip, peeled and cut into 1-inch chunks
- 1 tablespoon butter, melted
- 2 tablespoons honey
- 1 tablespoon dried parsley flakes, crushed
- ¼ teaspoon red pepper flakes, crushed
- Salt and ground black pepper, to taste

Directions:

1. Preheat the Air fryer to 355 °F and grease an Air fryer basket.
2. Mix the parsnips and butter in a bowl and toss to coat well.
3. Arrange the parsnip chunks in the Air fryer basket and cook for about 40 minutes.
4. Mix the remaining ingredients in another large bowl and stir in the parsnip chunks.
5. Transfer the parsnip chunks in the Air fryer basket and cook for about 4 minutes.
6. Dish out the parsnip chunks onto serving plates and serve hot.

97. Caribbean-style Fried Plantains

Servings: 2
Cooking Time: 20 Minutes
Ingredients:

- 2 plantains, peeled and cut into slices
- 2 tablespoons avocado oil
- 2 teaspoons Caribbean Sorrel Rum Spice Mix

Directions:

1. Toss the plantains with the avocado oil and spice mix.
2. Cook in the preheated Air Fryer at 400 degrees F for 10 minutes, shaking the cooking basket halfway through the cooking time.
3. Adjust the seasonings to taste and enjoy!

98. Cheddar, Squash 'n Zucchini Casserole

Servings:4
Cooking Time: 30 Minutes
Ingredients:

- 1 egg
- 5 saltine crackers, or as needed, crushed
- 2 tablespoons bread crumbs
- 1/2-pound yellow squash, sliced
- 1/2-pound zucchini, sliced
- 1/2 cup shredded Cheddar cheese
- 1-1/2 teaspoons white sugar
- 1/2 teaspoon salt
- 1/4 onion, diced
- 1/4 cup biscuit baking mix
- 1/4 cup butter

Directions:

1. Lightly grease baking pan of air fryer with cooking spray. Add onion, zucchini, and yellow squash. Cover pan with foil and for 15 minutes, cook on 360°F or until tender.
2. Stir in salt, sugar, egg, butter, baking mix, and cheddar cheese. Mix well. Fold in crushed crackers. Top with bread crumbs.
3. Cook for 15 minutes at 390°F until tops are lightly browned.
4. Serve and enjoy.

99. Baked Green Beans

Servings:6
Cooking Time: 20 Minutes
Ingredients:

- 2 whole eggs, beaten
- ½ cup Parmesan cheese, grated
- ½ cup flour
- 1 tsp cayenne pepper
- 1 ½ pounds green beans
- Salt to taste

Directions:

1. Preheat your air fryer to 400 F, and in a bowl, mix panko, Parmesan cheese, cayenne pepper, season with salt and pepper. Cover the green beans in flour and dip in eggs.
2. Dredge beans in the Parmesan-panko mix. Place the prepared beans in your air fryer's cooking basket and cook for 15 minutes. Serve

100.Vegetable Spring Rolls

Servings:4
Cooking Time: 15 Minutes
Ingredients:

- 2 carrots, grated
- 1 tsp minced ginger
- 1 tsp minced garlic
- 1 tsp sesame oil
- 1 tsp soy sauce
- 1 tsp sesame seeds
- ½ tsp salt
- 1 tsp olive oil

- 1 package spring roll wrappers

Directions:

1. Preheat the air fryer to 370 F, and combine all ingredients in a large bowl. Divide the mixture between the spring roll sheets, and roll them up; arrange on the baking mat. Cook in the air fryer for 5 minutes.

101.Traditional Indian Bhaji

Servings: 4
Cooking Time: 40 Minutes
Ingredients:

- 2 eggs, beaten
- 1/2 cup almond meal
- 1/2 cup coconut flour
- 1/2 teaspoon baking powder
- 1 teaspoon curry paste
- 1 teaspoon cumin seed
- 1 teaspoon minced fresh ginger root
- Salt and black pepper, to your liking
- 2 red onions, chopped
- 1 Indian green chili, pureed
- Non-stick cooking spray

Directions:

1. Whisk the eggs, almond meal, coconut flour and baking powder in a mixing dish to make a thick batter; add in the cold water if needed.
2. Add in curry paste, cumin seeds, ginger root, salt, and black pepper.
3. Now, add onions and chili pepper; mix until everything is well incorporated.
4. Shape the balls and slightly press them to make the patties. Spritz the patties with cooking oil on all sides.
5. Place a sheet of aluminum foil in the Air Fryer food basket. Place the fritters on foil.

6. Then, air-fry them at 360 degrees F for 15 minutes; flip them over, press the power button and cook for another 20 minutes. Serve right away!

102.Parsley-loaded Mushrooms

Servings:2
Cooking Time: 15 Minutes
Ingredients:

- 2 slices white bread
- 1 garlic clove, crushed
- 2 tsp olive oil
- 2 tbsp parsley, finely chopped
- salt and black pepper

Directions:

1. Preheat air fryer to 360 F. In a food processor, grind the bread into crumbs. Add garlic, parsley and pepper; mix and stir in the olive oil. Cut off the mushroom stalks and fill the caps with the breadcrumbs. Place the mushroom caps in the air fryer basket Cook for 10 minutes or until golden and crispy.

103.Herbed Eggplant

Servings:2
Cooking Time:15 Minutes
Ingredients:

- 1 large eggplant, cubed
- ½ teaspoon dried marjoram, crushed
- ½ teaspoon dried oregano, crushed
- ½ teaspoon dried thyme, crushed
- ½ teaspoon garlic powder
- Salt and black pepper, to taste
- Olive oil cooking spray

Directions:

1. Preheat the Air fryer to 390 °F and grease an Air fryer basket.
2. Mix herbs, garlic powder, salt, and black pepper in a bowl.

3. Spray the eggplant cubes with cooking spray and rub with the herb mixture.
4. Arrange the eggplant cubes in the Air fryer basket and cook for about 15 minutes, flipping twice in between.
5. Dish out onto serving plates and serve hot.

104.Crispy Marinated Tofu

Servings:3
Cooking Time: 20 Minutes
Ingredients:
- 1 (14-ounces) block firm tofu, pressed and cut into 1-inch cubes
- 2 tablespoons low sodium soy sauce
- 2 teaspoons sesame oil, toasted
- 1 teaspoon seasoned rice vinegar
- 1 tablespoon cornstarch

Directions:
1. In a bowl, mix well tofu, soy sauce, sesame oil, and vinegar.
2. Set aside to marinate for about 25-30 minutes.
3. Coat the tofu cubes evenly with cornstarch.
4. Set the temperature of air fryer to 370 degrees F. Grease an air fryer basket.
5. Arrange tofu pieces into the prepared air fryer basket in a single layer.
6. Air fry for about 20 minutes, shaking once halfway through.
7. Remove from air fryer and transfer the tofu onto serving plates.
8. Serve warm.

105.Air-fried Cauliflower

Servings:4
Cooking Time: 20 Minutes
Ingredients:
- 2 tbsp olive oil

- ½ tsp salt
- ¼ tsp freshly ground black pepper

Directions:
1. In a bowl, toss cauliflower, oil, salt, and black pepper, until the florets are well-coated. Arrange the florets in the air fryer and cook for 8 minutes at 360 F; work in batches if needed. Serve the crispy cauliflower in lettuce wraps with chicken, cheese or mushrooms.

106.Ooey-gooey Dessert Quesadilla

Servings: 2
Cooking Time: 25 Minutes
Ingredients:
- 1/4 cup blueberries
- 1/4 cup fresh orange juice
- 1/2 tablespoon maple syrup
- 1/2 cup vegan cream cheese
- 1 teaspoon vanilla extract
- 2 (6-inch tortillas
- 2 teaspoons coconut oil
- 1/4 cup vegan dark chocolate

Directions:
1. Bring the blueberries, orange juice, and maple syrup to a boil in a saucepan. Reduce the heat and let it simmer until the sauce thickens, about 10 minutes.
2. In a mixing dish, combine the cream cheese with the vanilla extract; spread on the tortillas. Add the blueberry filling on top. Fold in half.
3. Place the quesadillas in the greased Air Fryer basket. Cook at 390 degrees F for 10 minutes, until tortillas are golden brown and filling is melted. Make sure to turn them over halfway through the cooking.

4. Heat the coconut oil in a small pan and add the chocolate; whisk to combine well. Drizzle the chocolate sauce over the quesadilla and serve. Enjoy!

107.Air Fried Vegetables With Garlic

Servings:6
Cooking Time: 25 Minutes
Ingredients:
- ¾ lb tomatoes
- 1 medium onion
- 1 tbsp lemon juice
- 1 tbsp olive oil
- ½ tbsp salt
- 1 tbsp coriander powder

Directions:
1. Preheat air fryer to 360 F. Place peppers, tomatoes, and onion in the basket. Cook for 5 minutes, then flip and cook for 5 more minutes. Remove and peel the skin. Place the vegetables in a blender and sprinkle with the salt and coriander powder. Blend to smooth and season with salt and olive oil.

108.Paprika Brussels Sprout Chips

Servings: 2
Cooking Time: 20 Minutes
Ingredients:
- 10 Brussels sprouts
- 1 teaspoon canola oil
- 1 teaspoon coarse sea salt
- 1 teaspoon paprika

Directions:
1. Toss all ingredients in the lightly greased Air Fryer basket.
2. Bake at 380 degrees F for 15 minutes, shaking the basket halfway through the cooking time to ensure even cooking.

3. Serve and enjoy!

109.Pesto Tomatoes

Servings:4
Cooking Time: 16 Minutes
Ingredients:
- For Pesto:
- ½ cup plus 1 tablespoon olive oil, divided
- 3 tablespoons pine nuts
- Salt, to taste
- ½ cup fresh basil, chopped
- ½ cup fresh parsley, chopped
- 1 garlic clove, chopped
- ½ cup Parmesan cheese, grated
- For Tomatoes:
- 2 heirloom tomatoes, cut into ½ inch thick slices
- 8 ounces feta cheese, cut into ½ inch thick slices.
- ½ cup red onions, thinly sliced
- 1 tablespoon olive oil
- Salt, to taste

Directions:
1. Set the temperature of air fryer to 390 degrees F. Grease an air fryer basket.
2. In a bowl, mix together one tablespoon of oil, pine nuts and pinch of salt.
3. Arrange pine nuts into the prepared air fryer basket.
4. Air fry for about 1-2 minutes.
5. Remove from air fryer and transfer the pine nuts onto a paper towel-lined plate.
6. In a food processor, add the toasted pine nuts, fresh herbs, garlic, Parmesan, and salt and pulse until just combined.

7. While motor is running, slowly add the remaining oil and pulse until smooth.
8. Transfer into a bowl, covered and refrigerate until serving.
9. Spread about one tablespoon of pesto onto each tomato slice.
10. Top each tomato slice with one feta and onion slice and drizzle with oil.
11. Arrange tomato slices into the prepared air fryer basket in a single layer.
12. Air fry for about 12-14 minutes.
13. Remove from air fryer and transfer the tomato slices onto serving plates.
14. Sprinkle with a little salt and serve with the remaining pesto.

110.Fried Falafel Recipe From The Middle East

Servings:8
Cooking Time: 15 Minutes
Ingredients:
- ¼ cup coriander, chopped
- ¼ cup parsley, chopped
- ½ onion, diced
- ½ teaspoon coriander seeds
- ½ teaspoon red pepper flakes
- ½ teaspoon salt
- 1 tablespoon juice from freshly squeezed lemon
- 1 teaspoon cumin seeds
- 2 cups chickpeas from can, drained and rinsed
- 3 cloves garlic
- 3 tablespoons all-purpose flour
- cooking spray

Directions:
1. In a skillet over medium heat, toast the cumin and coriander seeds until fragrant.
2. Place the toasted seeds in a mortar and grind the seeds.
3. In a food processor, place all ingredients except for the cooking spray. Add the toasted cumin and coriander seeds.
4. Pulse until fine.
5. Shape the mixture into falafels and spray cooking oil.
6. Place inside a preheated air fryer and make sure that they do not overlap.
7. Cook at 400 °F for 15 minutes or until the surface becomes golden brown.

111.Spicy Braised Vegetables

Servings: 4
Cooking Time: 25 Minutes
Ingredients:
- 1 large-sized zucchini, sliced
- 1 Serrano pepper, deveined and thinly sliced
- 2 bell peppers, deveined and thinly sliced
- 1 celery stalk, cut into matchsticks
- 1/4 cup olive oil
- 1/2 teaspoon porcini powder
- 1/4 teaspoon mustard powder
- 1/2 teaspoon fennel seeds
- 1 tablespoon garlic powder
- 1/2 teaspoon fine sea salt
- 1/4 teaspoon ground black pepper
- 1/2 cup tomato puree

Directions:
1. Place the sweet potatoes, zucchini, peppers, and the carrot into the Air Fryer cooking basket.
2. Drizzle with olive oil and toss to coat; cook in the preheated Air Fryer at 350 degrees F for 15 minutes.
3. While the vegetables are cooking, prepare the sauce by thoroughly

whisking the other ingredients, without the tomato ketchup. Lightly grease a baking dish that fits into your machine.

4. Transfer cooked vegetables to the prepared baking dish; add the sauce and toss to coat well.

5. Turn the Air Fryer to 390 degrees F and cook the vegetables for 5 more minutes. Bon appétit!

112.Swiss Cheese And Eggplant Crisps

Servings: 4
Cooking Time: 45 Minutes
Ingredients:

- 1/2 pound eggplant, sliced
- 1/4 cup almond meal
- 2 tablespoons flaxseed meal
- Coarse sea salt and ground black pepper, to taste
- 1 teaspoon paprika
- 1 cup parmesan, freshly grated

Directions:

1. Toss the eggplant with 1 tablespoon of salt and let it stand for 30 minutes. Drain and rinse well.

2. Mix the almond meal, flaxseed meal, salt, black pepper, and paprika in a bowl. Then, pour in the water and whisk to combine well.

3. Then, place parmesan in another shallow bowl.

4. Dip the eggplant slices in the almond meal mixture, then in parmesan; press to coat on all sides. Transfer to the lightly greased Air Fryer basket.

5. Cook at 370 degrees F for 6 minutes. Turn each slice over and cook an additional 5 minutes.

6. Serve garnished with spicy ketchup if desired. Bon appétit!

113.Sweet Potato French Fries

Servings:4
Cooking Time: 30 Minutes
Ingredients:

- ½ tsp garlic powder
- ½ tsp chili powder
- ¼ tsp cumin
- 3 tbsp olive oil
- 3 sweet potatoes, cut into thick strips

Directions:

1. In a bowl, mix salt, garlic powder, chili powder, and cumin, and whisk in oil. Coat the strips well in this mixture and arrange them on the air fryer's basket. Cook for 20 minutes at 380 F until crispy. Serve.

114.Herbed Carrots

Servings:8
Cooking Time:14 Minutes
Ingredients:

- 6 large carrots, peeled and sliced lengthwise
- 2 tablespoons olive oil
- ½ tablespoon fresh oregano, chopped
- ½ tablespoon fresh parsley, chopped
- Salt and black pepper, to taste
- 2 tablespoons olive oil, divided
- ½ cup fat-free Italian dressing
- Salt, to taste

Directions:

1. Preheat the Air fryer to 360 °F and grease an Air fryer basket.

2. Mix the carrot slices and olive oil in a bowl and toss to coat well.

3. Arrange the carrot slices in the Air fryer basket and cook for about 12 minutes.

4. Dish out the carrot slices onto serving plates and sprinkle with herbs, salt and black pepper.

5. Transfer into the Air fryer basket and cook for 2 more minutes.
6. Dish out and serve hot.

115.Sesame Seeds Bok Choy(1)

Servings:4
Cooking Time:6 Minutes
Ingredients:
- 4 bunches baby bok choy, bottoms removed and leaves separated
- 1 teaspoon sesame seeds
- Olive oil cooking spray
- 1 teaspoon garlic powder

Directions:
1. Preheat the Air fryer to 325 °F and grease an Air fryer basket.
2. Arrange the bok choy leaves into the Air fryer basket and spray with the cooking spray.
3. Sprinkle with garlic powder and cook for about 6 minutes, shaking twice in between.
4. Dish out in the bok choy onto serving plates and serve garnished with sesame seeds.

116.Cheese Pizza With Broccoli Crust

Servings: 1
Cooking Time: 30 Minutes
Ingredients:
- 3 cups broccoli rice, steamed
- ½ cup parmesan cheese, grated
- 1 egg
- 3 tbsp. low-carb Alfredo sauce
- ½ cup parmesan cheese, grated

Directions:
1. Drain the broccoli rice and combine with the parmesan cheese and egg in a bowl, mixing well.
2. Cut a piece of parchment paper roughly the size of the base of the fryer's basket. Spoon four equal-sized amounts of the broccoli mixture onto the paper and press each portion into the shape of a pizza crust. You may have to complete this part in two batches. Transfer the parchment to the fryer.
3. Cook at 370°F for five minutes. When the crust is firm, flip it over and cook for an additional two minutes.
4. Add the Alfredo sauce and mozzarella cheese on top of the crusts and cook for an additional seven minutes. The crusts are ready when the sauce and cheese have melted. Serve hot.

117.Easy Glazed Carrots

Servings:4
Cooking Time:12 Minutes
Ingredients:
- 3 cups carrots, peeled and cut into large chunks
- 1 tablespoon olive oil
- 1 tablespoon honey
- Salt and black pepper, to taste

Directions:
1. Preheat the Air fryer to 390 °F and grease an Air fryer basket.
2. Mix all the ingredients in a bowl and toss to coat well.
3. Transfer into the Air fryer basket and cook for about 12 minutes.
4. Dish out and serve hot.

118.Hungarian Mushroom Pilaf

Servings: 4
Cooking Time: 50 Minutes
Ingredients:
- 1 ½ cups white rice
- 3 cups vegetable broth
- 2 tablespoons olive oil
- 1 pound fresh porcini mushrooms, sliced

- 2 tablespoons olive oil
- 2 garlic cloves
- 1 onion, chopped
- 1/4 cup dry vermouth
- 1 teaspoon dried thyme
- 1/2 teaspoon dried tarragon
- 1 teaspoon sweet Hungarian paprika

Directions:

1. Place the rice and broth in a large saucepan, add water; and bring to a boil. Cover, turn the heat down to low, and continue cooking for 16 to 18 minutes more. Set aside for 5 to 10 minutes.
2. Now, stir the hot cooked rice with the remaining ingredients in a lightly greased baking dish.
3. Cook in the preheated Air Fryer at 370 degrees for 20 minutes, checking periodically to ensure even cooking.
4. Serve in individual bowls. Bon appétit!

119.Crispy Asparagus Dipped In Paprika-garlic Spice

Servings:5
Cooking Time:15 Minutes
Ingredients:

- ¼ cup almond flour
- ½ teaspoon garlic powder
- ½ teaspoon smoked paprika
- 10 medium asparagus, trimmed
- 2 large eggs, beaten
- 2 tablespoons parsley, chopped
- Salt and pepper to taste

Directions:

1. Preheat the air fryer for 5 minutes.
2. In a mixing bowl, combine the parsley, garlic powder, almond flour, and smoked paprika. Season with salt and pepper to taste.

3. Soak firs the asparagus in the beaten eggs and dredge in the almond flour mixture.
4. Place in the air fryer basket. Close.
5. Cook for 15 minutes at 350 °F.

120.Green Beans & Mushroom Casserole

Servings:6
Cooking Time: 12 Minutes
Ingredients:

- 24 ounces fresh green beans, trimmed
- 2 cups fresh button mushrooms, sliced
- 3 tablespoons olive oil
- 2 tablespoons fresh lemon juice
- 1 teaspoon ground sage
- 1 teaspoon garlic powder
- 1 teaspoon onion powder
- Salt and ground black pepper, as required
- 1/3 cup French fried onions*

Directions:

1. In a bowl, add the green beans, mushrooms, oil, lemon juice, sage, and spices and toss to coat well.
2. Set the temperature of air fryer to 400 degrees F. Lightly, grease an air fryer basket.
3. Arrange mushroom mixture into the prepared air fryer basket.
4. Air fry for about 10-12 minutes, shaking several times while frying.
5. Remove from air fryer and transfer the mushroom mixture into a serving dish.
6. Top with fried onions and serve.

121.Spicy Ricotta Stuffed Mushrooms

Servings: 4
Cooking Time: 25 Minutes
Ingredients:

- 1 pound small white mushrooms
- Sea salt and ground black pepper, to taste
- 4 tablespoons Ricotta cheese
- 1/2 teaspoon ancho chili powder
- 1 teaspoon paprika
- 1 egg
- 1/2 cup parmesan cheese, grated

Directions:

1. Remove the stems from the mushroom caps and chop them; mix the chopped mushrooms steams with the salt, black pepper, cheese, chili powder, and paprika.
2. Add in eggs and mix to combine well. Stuff the mushroom caps with the egg/cheese filling.
3. To with parmesan cheese. Spritz the stuffed mushrooms with cooking spray.
4. Cook in the preheated Air Fryer at 360 degrees F for 18 minutes. Bon appétit!

122.Crispy Butternut Squash Fries

Servings: 4
Cooking Time: 25 Minutes
Ingredients:

- 1 cup all-purpose flour
- Salt and ground black pepper, to taste
- 3 tablespoons nutritional yeast flakes
- 1/2 cup almond milk
- 1/2 cup almond meal
- 1/2 cup bread crumbs
- 1 tablespoon herbs (oregano, basil, rosemary, chopped)
- 1 pound butternut squash, peeled and cut into French fry shapes

Directions:

1. In a shallow bowl, combine the flour, salt, and black pepper. In another shallow dish, mix the nutritional yeast flakes with the almond milk until well combined.
2. Mix the almond meal, breadcrumbs, and herbs in a third shallow dish. Dredge the butternut squash in the flour mixture, shaking off the excess. Then, dip in the milk mixture; lastly, dredge in the breadcrumb mixture.
3. Spritz the butternut squash fries with cooking oil on all sides.
4. Cook in the preheated Air Fryer at 400 degrees F approximately 12 minutes, turning them over halfway through the cooking time.
5. Serve with your favorite sauce for dipping. Bon appétit!

123.Baby Corn In Chili-turmeric Spice

Servings:5
Cooking Time: 8 Minutes
Ingredients:

- ¼ cup water
- ¼ teaspoon baking soda
- ¼ teaspoon salt
- ¼ teaspoon turmeric powder
- ½ teaspoon curry powder
- ½ teaspoon red chili powder
- 1 cup chickpea flour or besan
- 10 pieces baby corn, blanched

Directions:

1. Preheat the air fryer to 400 °F.
2. Line the air fryer basket with aluminum foil and brush with oil.
3. In a mixing bowl, mix all ingredients except for the corn.
4. Whisk until well combined.
5. Dip the corn in the batter and place inside the air fryer. Cook for 8 minutes until golden brown.

124.Cheesy Bbq Tater Tot

Servings:6
Cooking Time: 20 Minutes

Ingredients:

- ½ cup shredded Cheddar
- 12 slices bacon
- 1-lb frozen tater tots, defrosted
- 2 tbsp chives
- Ranch dressing, for serving

Directions:

1. Thread one end of bacon in a skewer, followed by one tater, snuggly thread the bacon around tater like a snake, and then another tater, and then snake the bacon again until you reach the end. Repeat with the rest of the Ingredients.
2. For 10 minutes, cook on 360°F. Halfway through cooking time, turnover skewers. If needed cook in batches.
3. Place skewers on a serving platter and sprinkle cheese and chives on top.
4. Serve and enjoy with ranch dressing on the side.

POULTRY RECIPES

125.Broccoli-rice 'n Chees Casserole

Servings:4
Cooking Time: 28 Minutes
Ingredients:
- 1 (10 ounce) can chunk chicken, drained
- 1 cup uncooked instant rice
- 1 cup water
- 1/2 (10.75 ounce) can condensed cream of chicken soup
- 1/2 (10.75 ounce) can condensed cream of mushroom soup
- 1/2 cup milk
- 1/2 small white onion, chopped
- 1/2-pound processed cheese food
- 2 tablespoons butter
- 8-ounce frozen chopped broccoli

Directions:
1. Lightly grease baking pan of air fryer with cooking spray. Add water and bring to a boil at 390°F. Stir in rice and cook for 3 minutes.
2. Stir in processed cheese, onion, broccoli, milk, butter, chicken soup, mushroom soup, and chicken. Mix well.
3. Cook for 15 minutes at 390°F, fluff mixture and continue cooking for another 10 minutes until tops are browned.
4. Serve and enjoy.

126.Kung Pao Chicken

Servings: 4
Cooking Time: 50 Minutes
Ingredients:
- 1 ½ pounds chicken breast, halved
- 1 tablespoon lemon juice
- 2 tablespoons mirin
- 1/4 cup milk
- 2 tablespoons soy sauce
- 1 tablespoon olive oil
- 1 teaspoon ginger, peeled and grated
- 2 garlic cloves, minced
- 1/2 teaspoon salt
- 1/2 teaspoon Szechuan pepper
- 1/2 teaspoon xanthan gum

Directions:
1. In a large ceramic dish, place the chicken, lemon juice, mirin, milk, soy sauce, olive oil, ginger, and garlic. Let it marinate for 30 minutes in your refrigerator.
2. Spritz the sides and bottom of the cooking basket with a nonstick cooking spray. Arrange the chicken in the cooking basket and cook at 370 degrees F for 10 minutes.
3. Turn over the chicken, baste with the reserved marinade and cook for 4 minutes longer. Taste for doneness, season with salt and pepper, and reserve.
4. Add the marinade to the preheated skillet over medium heat; add in xanthan gum. Let it cook for 5 to 6 minutes until the sauce thickens.
5. Spoon the sauce over the reserved chicken and serve immediately.

127.Marinated Chicken Drumettes With Asparagus

Servings: 6
Cooking Time: 30 Minutes + Marinating Time
Ingredients:
- 6 chicken drumettes
- 1 ½ pounds asparagus, ends trimmed
- Marinade:
- 3 tablespoons canola oil

- 3 tablespoons soy sauce
- 3 tablespoons lime juice
- 3 heaping tablespoons shallots, minced
- 1 heaping teaspoon fresh garlic, minced
- 1 (1-inch piece fresh ginger, peeled and minced
- 1 teaspoon Creole seasoning
- Coarse sea salt and ground black pepper, to taste

Directions:

1. In a ceramic bowl, mix all ingredients for the marinade. Add the chicken drumettes and let them marinate at least 5 hours in the refrigerator.
2. Now, drain the chicken drumettes and discard the marinade.
3. Cook in the preheated Air Fryer at 370 degrees F for 11 minutes. Turn the chicken drumettes over and cook for a further 11 minutes.
4. While the chicken drumettes are cooking, add the reserved marinade to the preheated skillet. Add the asparagus and cook for approximately 5 minutes or until cooked through. Serve with the air-fried chicken and enjoy!

128.Sweet And Sour Chicken Thighs

Servings:2
Cooking Time:20 Minutes
Ingredients:

- 1 scallion, finely chopped
- 2 (4-ounces) skinless, boneless chicken thighs
- ½ cup corn flour
- 1 garlic clove, minced
- ½ tablespoon soy sauce
- ½ tablespoon rice vinegar

- 1 teaspoon sugar
- Salt and black pepper, as required

Directions:

1. Preheat the Air fryer to 390 °F and grease an Air fryer basket.
2. Mix all the ingredients except chicken and corn flour in a bowl.
3. Place the corn flour in another bowl.
4. Coat the chicken thighs into the marinade and then dredge into the corn flour.
5. Arrange the chicken thighs into the Air Fryer basket, skin side down and cook for about 10 minutes.
6. Set the Air fryer to 355 °F and cook for 10 more minutes.
7. Dish out the chicken thighs onto a serving platter and serve hot.

129.Flavorful Fried Chicken

Servings: 10
Cooking Time: 40 Minutes
Ingredients:

- 5 lbs chicken, about 10 pieces
- 1 tbsp coconut oil
- 2 1/2 tsp white pepper
- 1 tsp ground ginger
- 1 1/2 tsp garlic salt
- 1 tbsp paprika
- 1 tsp dried mustard
- 1 tsp pepper
- 1 tsp celery salt
- 1/3 tsp oregano
- 1/2 tsp basil
- 1/2 tsp thyme
- 2 cups pork rinds, crushed
- 1 tbsp vinegar
- 1 cup unsweetened almond milk
- 1/2 tsp salt

Directions:

1. Add chicken in a large mixing bowl.

2. Add milk and vinegar over chicken and place in the refrigerator for 2 hours.
3. I a shallow dish, mix together pork rinds, white pepper, ginger, garlic salt, paprika, mustard, pepper, celery salt, oregano, basil, thyme, and salt.
4. Coat air fryer basket with coconut oil.
5. Coat each chicken piece with pork rind mixture and place on a plate.
6. Place half coated chicken in the air fryer basket.
7. Cook chicken at 360 F for 10 minutes then turn chicken to another side and cook for 10 minutes more or until internal temperature reaches at 165 F.
8. Cook remaining chicken using the same method.
9. Serve and enjoy.

130.Traditional Chicken Teriyaki

Servings: 4
Cooking Time: 50 Minutes
Ingredients:
- 1 ½ pounds chicken breast, halved
- 1 tablespoon lemon juice
- 2 tablespoons Mirin
- 1/4 cup milk
- 2 tablespoons soy sauce
- 1 tablespoon olive oil
- 1 teaspoon ginger, peeled and grated
- 2 garlic cloves, minced
- 1/2 teaspoon salt
- 1/2 teaspoon ground black pepper
- 1 teaspoon cornstarch

Directions:
1. In a large ceramic dish, place the chicken, lemon juice, Mirin, milk, soy sauce, olive oil, ginger, and garlic. Let

it marinate for 30 minutes in your refrigerator.
2. Spritz the sides and bottom of the cooking basket with a nonstick cooking spray. Arrange the chicken in the cooking basket and cook at 370 degrees F for 10 minutes.
3. Turn over the chicken, baste with the reserved marinade and cook for 4 minutes longer. Taste for doneness, season with salt and pepper, and reserve.
4. Mix the cornstarch with 1 tablespoon of water. Add the marinade to the preheated skillet over medium heat; cook for 3 to 4 minutes. Now, stir in the cornstarch slurry and cook until the sauce thickens.
5. Spoon the sauce over the reserved chicken and serve immediately.

131.Cornish Game Hens

Servings:4
Cooking Time:16 Minutes
Ingredients:
- 1 teaspoon fresh rosemary, chopped
- 1 teaspoon fresh thyme, chopped
- 2 pounds Cornish game hen, backbone removed and halved
- ½ cup olive oil
- ¼ teaspoon sugar
- ¼ teaspoon red pepper flakes, crushed
- Salt and black pepper, to taste
- 1 teaspoon fresh lemon zest, finely grated

Directions:
1. Preheat the Air fryer to 390 °F and grease an Air fryer basket.
2. Mix olive oil, herbs, lemon zest, sugar, and spices in a bowl.

3. Stir in the Cornish game hen and refrigerate to marinate well for about 24 hours.
4. Transfer the Cornish game hen to the Air fryer and cook for about 16 minutes.
5. Dish out the hen portions onto serving plates and serve hot.

132.Cilantro-lime 'n Liquid Smoke Chicken Grill

Servings:4
Cooking Time: 40 Minutes
Ingredients:
- 1 ½ teaspoon honey
- 1 tablespoon lime zest
- 1 teaspoon liquid smoke
- 1/3 cup chopped cilantro
- 1/3 cup fresh lime juice
- 2 tablespoons olive oil
- 3 cloves of garlic, minced
- 4 chicken breasts, halved
- Salt and pepper to taste

Directions:
1. Place all Ingredients in a bowl and allow to marinate in the fridge for at least 2 hours.
2. Preheat the air fryer to 390 °F.
3. Place the grill pan accessory in the air fryer.
4. Grill in the chicken for 40 minutes and make sure to flip the chicken every 10 minutes for even grilling.

133.Chicken Popcorn

Servings: 6
Cooking Time: 10 Minutes
Ingredients:
- 4 eggs
- 1 1/2 lbs chicken breasts, cut into small chunks
- 1 tsp paprika

- 1/2 tsp garlic powder
- 1 tsp onion powder
- 2 1/2 cups pork rind, crushed
- 1/4 cup coconut flour
- Pepper
- Salt

Directions:
1. In a small bowl, mix together coconut flour, pepper, and salt.
2. In another bowl, whisk eggs until combined.
3. Take one more bowl and mix together pork panko, paprika, garlic powder, and onion powder.
4. Add chicken pieces in a large mixing bowl. Sprinkle coconut flour mixture over chicken and toss well.
5. Dip chicken pieces in the egg mixture and coat with pork panko mixture and place on a plate.
6. Spray air fryer basket with cooking spray.
7. Preheat the air fryer to 400 F.
8. Add half prepared chicken in air fryer basket and cook for 10-12 minutes. Shake basket halfway through.
9. Cook remaining half using the same method.
10. Serve and enjoy.

134.Coconut Turkey And Spinach Mix

Servings: 4
Cooking Time: 15 Minutes
Ingredients:
- 1 pound turkey meat, ground and browned
- 1 tablespoon garlic, minced
- 1 tablespoon ginger, grated
- 2 tablespoons coconut aminos
- 4 cups spinach leaves
- A pinch of salt and black pepper

Directions:
1. In a pan that fits your air fryer, combine all the ingredients and toss. Put the pan in the air fryer and cook at 380 degrees F for 15 minutes Divide everything into bowls and serve.

135.Air Fried Southern Drumsticks

Servings:4
Cooking Time: 50 Minutes
Ingredients:
- 2 tbsp oregano
- 2 tbsp thyme
- 2 oz oats
- ¼ cup milk
- ¼ steamed cauliflower florets
- 1 egg
- 1 tbsp ground cayenne
- Salt and pepper, to taste

Directions:
1. Preheat the air fryer to 350 F and season the drumsticks with salt and pepper; rub them with the milk. Place all the other ingredients, except the egg, in a food processor. Process until smooth.
2. Dip each drumstick in the egg first, and then in the oat mixture. Arrange half of them on a baking mat inside the air fryer. Cook for 20 minutes. Repeat with the other batch.

136.Caprese Chicken With Balsamic Sauce

Servings:6
Cooking Time: 25 Minutes
Ingredients:
- 6 basil leaves
- ¼ cup balsamic vinegar
- 6 slices tomato
- 1 tbsp butter
- 6 slices mozzarella cheese

Directions:
1. Preheat your Fryer to 400 F and heat butter and balsamic vinegar in a frying pan over medium heat. Cover the chicken meat with the marinade. Place the chicken in the cooking basket and cook for 20 minutes. Cover the chicken with basil, tomato slices and cheese. Serve and enjoy!

137.Dijon-garlic Thighs

Servings:6
Cooking Time: 25 Minutes
Ingredients:
- 1 tablespoon cider vinegar
- 1 tablespoon Dijon mustard
- 1-pound chicken thighs
- 2 tablespoon olive oil
- 2 teaspoons herbs de Provence
- Salt and pepper to taste

Directions:
1. Place all ingredients in a Ziploc bag.
2. Allow to marinate in the fridge for at least 2 hours.
3. Preheat the air fryer for 5 minutes.
4. Place the chicken in the fryer basket.
5. Cook for 25 minutes at 350 °F.

138.Chicken Breasts With Chimichurri

Servings:1
Cooking Time:35 Minutes
Ingredients:
- 1 chicken breast, bone-in, skin-on
- Chimichurri
- ½ bunch fresh cilantro
- 1/4 bunch fresh parsley
- ½ shallot, peeled, cut in quarters
- ½ tablespoon paprika ground
- ½ tablespoon chili powder
- ½ tablespoon fennel ground
- ½ teaspoon black pepper, ground

- ½ teaspoon onion powder
- 1 teaspoon salt
- ½ teaspoon garlic powder
- ½ teaspoon cumin ground
- ½ tablespoon canola oil
- Chimichurri
- 2 tablespoons olive oil
- 4 garlic cloves, peeled
- Zest and juice of 1 lemon
- 1 teaspoon kosher salt

Directions:
1. Preheat the Air fryer to 300 °F and grease an Air fryer basket.
2. Combine all the spices in a suitable bowl and season the chicken with it.
3. Sprinkle with canola oil and arrange the chicken in the Air fryer basket.
4. Cook for about 35 minutes and dish out in a platter.
5. Put all the ingredients in the blender and blend until smooth.
6. Serve the chicken with chimichurri sauce.

139.Curried Chicken

Servings:3
Cooking Time:18 Minutes
Ingredients:
- 1 pound boneless chicken, cubed
- ½ tablespoon cornstarch
- 1 egg
- 1 medium yellow onion, thinly sliced
- ½ cup evaporated milk
- 1 tablespoon light soy sauce
- 2 tablespoons olive oil
- 3 teaspoons garlic, minced
- 1 teaspoon fresh ginger, grated
- 5 curry leaves
- 1 teaspoon curry powder
- 1 tablespoon chili sauce
- 1 teaspoon sugar

- Salt and black pepper, as required

Directions:
1. Preheat the Air fryer to 390 °F and grease an Air fryer basket.
2. Mix the chicken cubes, soy sauce, cornstarch and egg in a bowl and keep aside for about 1 hour.
3. Arrange the chicken cubes into the Air Fryer basket and cook for about 10 minutes.
4. Heat olive oil in a medium skillet and add onion, green chili, garlic, ginger, and curry leaves.
5. Sauté for about 4 minutes and stir in the chicken cubes, curry powder, chili sauce, sugar, salt, and black pepper.
6. Mix well and add the evaporated milk.
7. Cook for about 4 minutes and dish out the chicken mixture into a serving bowl to serve.

140.Chestnuts 'n Mushroom Chicken Casserole

Servings:2
Cooking Time: 35 Minutes
Ingredients:
- 1 (10.75 ounce) can condensed cream of chicken soup
- 1 (4.5 ounce) can mushrooms, drained
- 1 1/2 teaspoons melted butter
- 1 cup shredded, cooked chicken meat
- 1/2 (8 ounce) can water chestnuts, drained (optional)
- 1/2 cup mayonnaise
- 1/2 teaspoon lemon juice
- 1/4 cup shredded Cheddar cheese
- 1/8 teaspoon curry powder
- 1-1/4 cups cooked chopped broccoli

Directions:

1. Lightly grease baking pan of air fryer with cooking spray.
2. Evenly spread broccoli on bottom of pan. Sprinkle chicken on top, followed by water chestnuts and mushrooms.
3. In a bowl, whisk well melted butter, curry powder, lemon juice, mayonnaise, and soup. Pour over chicken mixture in pan. Cover pan with foil.
4. For 25 minutes, cook on 360°F.
5. Remove foil from pan and cook for another 10 minutes or until top is a golden brown.
6. Serve and enjoy.

141. Curry Duck Mix

Servings: 4
Cooking Time: 25 Minutes
Ingredients:

- 15 ounces duck breasts, skinless, boneless and cubed
- 1 tablespoon olive oil
- 2 shallots, chopped
- Salt and black pepper to the taste
- 5 ounces heavy cream
- 1 teaspoon curry powder
- ½ bunch coriander, chopped

Directions:

1. Heat up a pan that fits your air fryer with the oil over medium heat, add the duck, toss and brown for 5 minutes. Add the rest of the ingredients, toss, introduce the pan in the air fryer and cook at 370 degrees F for 20 minutes. Divide the mix into bowls and serve.

142. Yummy Stuffed Chicken Breast

Servings: 4
Cooking Time: 15 Minutes

Ingredients:

- 2 (8-ounce) chicken fillets, skinless and boneless, each cut into 2 pieces
- 4 brie cheese slices
- 1 tablespoon chive, minced
- 4 cured ham slices
- Salt and black pepper, to taste

Directions:

1. Preheat the Air fryer to 355 °F and grease an Air fryer basket.
2. Make a slit in each chicken piece horizontally and season with the salt and black pepper.
3. Insert cheese slice in the slits and sprinkle with chives.
4. Wrap each chicken piece with one ham slice and transfer into the Air fryer basket.
5. Cook for about 15 minutes and dish out to serve warm.

143. Sesame Chicken Wings

Servings: 4
Cooking Time: 25 Minutes
Ingredients:

- 2 tbsp sesame oil
- 2 tbsp maple syrup
- Salt and black pepper
- 3 tbsp sesame seeds

Directions:

1. In a bowl, add wings, oil, maple syrup, salt and pepper, and stir to coat well. In another bowl, add the sesame seeds and roll the wings in the seeds to coat thoroughly. Arrange the wings in an even layer inside your air fryer and cook for 12 minutes on 360 F, turning once halfway through.

144. Pineapple Juice-soy Sauce Marinated Chicken

Servings: 5

Cooking Time: 20 Minutes

Ingredients:

- 3 tablespoons light soy sauce
- 1-pound chicken breast tenderloins or strips
- 1/2 cup pineapple juice
- 1/4 cup packed brown sugar

Directions:

1. In a small saucepan bring to a boil pineapple juice, brown sugar, and soy sauce. Transfer to a large bowl. Stir in chicken and pineapple. Let it marinate in the fridge for an hour.
2. Thread pineapple and chicken in skewers. Place on skewer rack.
3. For 10 minutes, cook on 360°F. Halfway through cooking time, turnover chicken and baste with marinade.
4. Serve and enjoy.

145.The Best Pizza Chicken Ever

Servings: 4

Cooking Time: 20 Minutes

Ingredients:

- 4 small-sized chicken breasts, boneless and skinless
- 1/4 cup pizza sauce
- 1/2 cup Colby cheese, shredded
- 16 slices pepperoni
- Salt and pepper, to savor
- 1 ½ tablespoons olive oil
- 1 ½ tablespoons dried oregano

Directions:

1. Carefully flatten out the chicken breast using a rolling pin.
2. Divide the ingredients among four chicken fillets. Roll the chicken fillets with the stuffing and seal them using a small skewer or two toothpicks.
3. Roast in the preheated Air Fryer grill pan for 13 to 15 minutes at 370 degrees F. Bon appétit!

146.Ground Turkey Mix

Servings: 4

Cooking Time: 25 Minutes

Ingredients:

- 1 pound turkey meat, ground
- A pinch of salt and black pepper
- 2 tablespoons olive oil
- 2 teaspoons parsley flakes
- 1 pound green beans, trimmed and halved
- 2 teaspoons garlic powder

Directions:

1. Heat up a pan that fits the air fryer with the oil over medium-high heat, add the meat and brown it for 5 minutes. Add the remaining ingredients, toss, put the pan in the machine and cook at 370 degrees F for 20 minutes. Divide between plates and serve.

147.Herbed Turkey Breast

Servings:3

Cooking Time:35 Minutes

Ingredients:

- 1 (2½-pounds) bone-in, skin-on turkey breast
- 1 teaspoon dried thyme, crushed
- 1 teaspoon dried rosemary, crushed
- ½ teaspoon dried sage, crushed
- ½ teaspoon dark brown sugar
- ½ teaspoon garlic powder
- ½ teaspoon paprika
- 1 tablespoon olive oil

Directions:

1. Preheat the Air fryer to 360 °F and grease an Air fryer basket.
2. Mix the herbs, brown sugar, and spices in a bowl.
3. Drizzle the turkey breast with oil and season with the herb mixture.
4. Arrange the turkey breast into the Air Fryer basket, skin side down and cook for about 35 minutes, flipping once in between.

5. Dish out in a platter and cut into desired size slices to serve.

148.Chicken With Veggies

Servings:2
Cooking Time:45 Minutes
Ingredients:
- 4 small artichoke hearts, quartered
- 4 fresh large button mushrooms, quartered
- ½ small onion, cut in large chunks
- 2 skinless, boneless chicken breasts
- 2 tablespoons fresh parsley, chopped
- 2 garlic cloves, minced
- 2 tablespoons chicken broth
- 2 tablespoons red wine vinegar
- 2 tablespoons olive oil
- 1 tablespoon Dijon mustard
- 1/8 teaspoon dried thyme
- 1/8 teaspoon dried basil
- Salt and black pepper, as required

Directions:
1. Preheat the Air fryer to 350 °F and grease a baking dish lightly.
2. Mix the garlic, broth, vinegar, olive oil, mustard, thyme, and basil in a bowl.
3. Place the artichokes, mushrooms, onions, salt, and black pepper in the baking dish.
4. Layer with the chicken breasts and spread half of the mustard mixture evenly on it.
5. Transfer the baking dish into the Air fryer basket and cook for about 23 minutes.
6. Coat the chicken breasts with the remaining mustard mixture and flip the side.
7. Cook for about 22 minutes and serve garnished with parsley.

149.Vinegar Chicken

Servings:4
Cooking Time: 15 Minutes
Ingredients:
- 16 oz chicken thighs, skinless

- 1 teaspoon ground celery root
- 1 teaspoon dried celery leaves
- 1 teaspoon apple cider vinegar
- ½ teaspoon salt
- 1 tablespoon sunflower oil

Directions:
1. Rub the chicken thighs with the celery root, dried celery leaves, and salt. Then sprinkle the chicken with apple cider vinegar and sunflower oil. Leave it for 15 minutes to marinate. After this, preheat the air fryer to 385F. Put the chicken thighs in the air fryer and cook them for 12 minutes. Then flip the chicken on another side and cook for 3 minutes more. Transfer the cooked chicken thighs on the plate.

150.Mesmerizing Honey Chicken Drumsticks

Servings:3
Cooking Time: 20 Minutes
Ingredients:
- 2 tbsp olive oil
- 2 tbsp honey
- ½ tbsp garlic, minced

Directions:
1. Preheat your air fryer to 400 F. Add garlic, oil and honey to a sealable zip bag. Add chicken and toss to coat; set aside for 30 minutes. Add the coated chicken to the air fryer basket, and cook for 15 minutes.

151.Crispy Chicken Wings

Servings:2
Cooking Time: 25 Minutes
Ingredients:
- 2 lemongrass stalk (white portion), minced
- 1 onion, finely chopped
- 1 tablespoon soy sauce
- 1½ tablespoons honey
- Salt and ground white pepper, as required

- 1 pound chicken wings, rinsed and trimmed
- ½ cup cornstarch

Directions:
1. In a bowl, mix together the lemongrass, onion, soy sauce, honey, salt, and white pepper.
2. Add the wings and generously coat with marinade.
3. Cover and refrigerate to marinate overnight.
4. Set the temperature of Air Fryer to 355 degrees F. Grease an Air Fryer basket.
5. Remove the chicken wings from marinade and coat with the cornstarch.
6. Arrange chicken wings into the prepared Air Fryer basket in a single layer.
7. Air Fry for about 25 minutes, flipping once halfway through.
8. Remove from Air Fryer and transfer the chicken wings onto a serving platter.
9. Serve hot.

152.Chicken And Brown Rice Bake

Servings: 3
Cooking Time: 50 Minutes
Ingredients:
- 1 cup brown rice
- 2 cups vegetable broth
- 1/2 cup water
- 1 tablespoon butter, melted
- 1 onion, chopped
- 2 garlic cloves, minced
- Kosher salt and ground black pepper, to taste
- 1 teaspoon cayenne pepper
- 3 chicken fillets
- 1 cup tomato puree
- 1 tablespoon fresh chives, chopped

Directions:
1. Heat the brown rice, vegetable broth and water in a pot over high heat.

Bring it to a boil; turn the stove down to simmer and cook for 35 minutes.
2. Grease a baking pan with butter.
3. Spoon the prepared rice mixture into the baking pan. Add the onion, garlic, salt, black pepper, cayenne pepper, and chicken. Spoon the tomato puree over the chicken.
4. Cook in the preheated Air Fryer at 380 degrees F for 12 minutes. Serve garnished with fresh chives. Enjoy!

153.Delicious Turkey Sandwiches

Servings: 4
Cooking Time: 45 Minutes
Ingredients:
- 1 pound turkey tenderloins
- 1 tablespoon Dijon-style mustard
- 1 tablespoon olive oil
- Sea salt and ground black pepper, to taste
- 1 teaspoon Italian seasoning mix
- 1/4 cup all-purpose flour
- 1 cup turkey stock
- 8 slices sourdough, toasted
- 4 tablespoons tomato ketchup
- 4 tablespoons mayonnaise
- 4 pickles, sliced

Directions:
1. Rub the turkey tenderloins with the mustard and olive oil. Season with salt, black pepper, and Italian seasoning mix.
2. Cook the turkey tenderloins at 350 degrees F for 30 minutes, flipping them over halfway through. Let them rest for 5 to 7 minutes before slicing.
3. For the gravy, in a saucepan, place the drippings from the roasted turkey. Add 1/8 cup of flour and 1/2 cup of turkey stock; whisk until it makes a smooth paste.
4. Once it gets a golden brown color, add the rest of the stock and flour. Season with salt to taste. Let it

simmer over medium heat, stirring constantly for 6 to 7 minutes.

5. Assemble the sandwiches with the turkey, gravy, tomato ketchup, mayonnaise, and pickles. Serve and enjoy!

154.Orange-tequila Glazed Chicken

Servings:6
Cooking Time: 40 Minutes
Ingredients:
- ¼ cup tequila
- 1 shallot, minced
- 1/3 cup orange juice
- 2 tablespoons brown sugar
- 2 tablespoons honey
- 2 tablespoons whole coriander seeds
- 3 cloves of garlic, minced
- 3 pounds chicken breasts
- Salt and pepper to taste

Directions:
1. Place all Ingredients in a Ziploc bag and allow to marinate for at least 2 hours in the fridge.
2. Preheat the air fryer to 390 °F.
3. Place the grill pan accessory in the air fryer.
4. Grill the chicken for at least 40 minutes
5. Flip the chicken every 10 minutes for even cooking.
6. Meanwhile, pour the marinade in a saucepan and simmer until the sauce thickens.

7. Brush the chicken with the glaze before serving.

155.Hot Peppery Turkey Sandwiches

Servings:4
Cooking Time:25 Minutes
Ingredients:
- 1 cup leftover turkey, cut into bite-sized chunks
- 2 bell peppers, deveined and chopped
- 1 Serrano pepper, deveined and chopped
- 1 leek, sliced
- 1/2 cup sour cream
- 1 teaspoon hot paprika
- 3/4 teaspoon kosher salt
- 1/2 teaspoon ground black pepper
- 1 heaping tablespoon fresh cilantro, chopped
- A few dashes of Tabasco sauce
- 4 hamburger buns

Directions:
1. Toss all ingredients, without the hamburger buns, in an Air Fryer baking pan; toss until everything is well coated.
2. Now, roast it for 20 minutes at 385 degrees F. Serve on hamburger buns; add some extra sour cream and Dijon mustard if desired. Bon appétit!

BEEF,PORK & LAMB RECIPES

156.Beef Taco Wraps

Servings:6

Cooking Time: 4 Minutes

Ingredients:

- 6 (12-inch) flour tortillas
- 2 pounds cooked ground beef
- 12 ounces nacho cheese
- 6 tostadas
- 2 cups sour cream
- 2 cups Bibb lettuce, shredded
- 3 Roma tomatoes, sliced
- 2 cups Mexican blend cheese, shredded
- Olive oil cooking spray

Directions:

1. Arrange the tortillas onto a smooth surface.
2. Divide each ingredient into 6 portions.
3. Place 1 portion of beef in the center of each tortilla, followed by the nacho cheese, tostada, sour cream, lettuce, tomato slices and Mexican cheese.
4. Bring the edges of each tortilla up, over the center to look like a pinwheel.
5. Set the temperature of Air Fryer to 400 degrees F. Grease an Air Fryer basket.
6. Arrange taco wraps into the prepared Air Fryer basket, seam side down and spray each with cooking spray.
7. Air Fry for about 2 minutes.
8. Carefully flip the wraps and spray each with cooking spray again.
9. Air Fry for about 2 more minutes.
10. Remove from Air Fryer and transfer the wraps onto a platter.
11. Serve warm.

157.Spicy Pork With Herbs And Candy Onions

Servings: 4

Cooking Time: 1 Hour

Ingredients:

- 1 rosemary sprig, chopped
- 1 thyme sprig, chopped
- 1 teaspoon dried sage, crushed
- Sea salt and ground black pepper, to taste
- 1 teaspoon cayenne pepper
- 2 teaspoons sesame oil
- 2 pounds pork leg roast, scored
- 1/2 pound candy onions, peeled
- 2 chili peppers, minced
- 4 cloves garlic, finely chopped

Directions:

1. Start by preheating your Air Fryer to 400 degrees F.
2. Then, mix the seasonings with the sesame oil.
3. Rub the seasoning mixture all over the pork leg. Cook in the preheated Air Fryer for 40 minutes.
4. Add the candy onions, peppers and garlic and cook an additional 12 minutes. Slice the pork leg. Afterwards, spoon the pan juices over the meat and serve with the candy onions. Bon appétit!

158.Shoulder Steak With Herbs And Brussels Sprouts

Servings: 4

Cooking Time: 30 Minutes + Marinating Time

Ingredients:

- 1 pound beef chuck shoulder steak
- 2 tablespoons vegetable oil
- 1 tablespoon red wine vinegar

- 1 teaspoon fine sea salt
- 1/2 teaspoon ground black pepper
- 1 teaspoon smoked paprika
- 1 teaspoon onion powder
- 1/2 teaspoon garlic powder
- 1/2 pound Brussels sprouts, cleaned and halved
- 1/2 teaspoon fennel seeds
- 1 teaspoon dried basil
- 1 teaspoon dried sage

Directions:

1. Firstly, marinate the beef with vegetable oil, wine vinegar, salt, black pepper, paprika, onion powder, and garlic powder. Rub the marinade into the meat and let it stay at least for 3 hours.
2. Air fry at 390 degrees F for 10 minutes. Pause the machine and add the prepared Brussels sprouts; sprinkle them with fennel seeds, basil, and sage.
3. Turn the machine to 380 degrees F; press the power button and cook for 5 more minutes. Pause the machine, stir and cook for further 10 minutes.
4. Next, remove the meat from the cooking basket and cook the vegetables a few minutes more if needed and according to your taste. Serve with your favorite mayo sauce.

159.Maras Pepper Lamb Kebab Recipe From Turkey

Servings:2
Cooking Time: 15 Minutes
Ingredients:

- 1-lb lamb meat, cut into 2-inch cubes
- Kosher salt
- Freshly cracked black pepper

- 2 tablespoons Maras pepper, or 2 teaspoons other dried chili powder mixed with 1 tablespoon paprika
- 1 teaspoon minced garlic
- 2 tablespoons roughly chopped fresh mint
- 1/2 cup extra-virgin olive oil, divided
- 1/2 cup dried apricots, cut into medium dice

Directions:

1. In a bowl, mix pepper, salt, and half of olive oil. Add lamb and toss well to coat. Thread lamb into 4 skewers.
2. Cook for 5 minutes at 390°F or to desired doneness.
3. In a large bowl, mix well remaining oil, mint, garlic, Maras pepper, and apricots. Add cooked lamb. Season with salt and pepper. Toss well to coat
4. Serve and enjoy.

160.Lamb With Olives

Servings: 4
Cooking Time: 35 Minutes
Ingredients:

- 1 and ½ pounds lamb meat, cubed
- 2 tablespoons olive oil
- A pinch of salt and black pepper
- ¼ cup kalamata olives, pitted and sliced
- 4 garlic cloves, minced
- Zest of 1 lemon, grated
- 2 rosemary springs, chopped
- 6 tomatoes, cubed

Directions:

1. Heat up a pan that fits your air fryer with the oil over medium heat, add the meat and brown for 5 minutes. Add the rest of the ingredients, toss, put the pan in the air fryer and cook

at 380 degrees F for 30 minutes. Divide everything into bowls and serve.

161.Greek Pork And Spinach

Servings: 4
Cooking Time: 25 Minutes
Ingredients:

- 2 pounds pork tenderloin, cut into strips
- 2 tablespoons coconut oil, melted
- A pinch of salt and black pepper
- 6 ounces baby spinach
- 1 cup cherry tomatoes, halved
- 1 cup feta cheese, crumbled

Directions:

1. Heat up a pan that fits your air fryer with the oil over medium high heat, add the pork and brown for 5 minutes. Add the rest of the ingredients except the spinach and the cheese, put the pan to your air fryer, cook at 390 degrees F for 15 minutes. Add the spinach, toss, and cook for 5 minutes more. Divide between plates and serve with feta cheese sprinkled on top.

162.Thyme And Turmeric Pork

Servings: 4
Cooking Time: 15 Minutes
Ingredients:

- 1-pound pork tenderloin
- ½ teaspoon salt
- ½ teaspoon ground turmeric
- 1 tablespoon dried thyme
- 1 tablespoon avocado oil

Directions:

1. Rub the pork tenderloin with salt, ground turmeric, and dried thyme. Then brush it with avocado oil. Preheat the air fryer to 370F. Place

the pork tenderloin in the air fryer basket and cook it for 15 minutes. You can flip the meat on another side during cooking if desired.

163.Spicy Pork Curry

Servings: 4
Cooking Time: 35 Minutes
Ingredients:

- 2 cardamom pods, only the seeds, crushed
- 1 teaspoon fennel seeds
- 1 teaspoon cumin seeds
- 1 teaspoon coriander seeds
- 2 teaspoons peanut oil
- 2 scallions, chopped
- 2 garlic cloves, smashed
- 2 jalapeno peppers, minced
- 1/2 teaspoon ginger, freshly grated
- 1 pound pork loin, cut into bite-sized cubes
- 1 cup coconut milk
- 1 cup chicken broth
- 1 teaspoon turmeric powder
- 1 tablespoon tamarind paste
- 1 tablespoon fresh lime juice

Directions:

1. Place the cardamom, fennel, cumin, and coriander seeds in a nonstick skillet over medium-high heat. Stir for 6 minutes until the spices become aromatic and start to brown. Stir frequently to prevent the spices from burning. Set aside.
2. Preheat your Air Fryer to 370 degrees F. Then, in a baking pan, heat the peanut oil for 2 minutes. Once hot, sauté the scallions for 2 to 3 minutes until tender.
3. Stir in the garlic, peppers, and ginger; cook an additional minute, stirring

frequently. Next, cook the pork for 3 to 4 minutes.

4. Pour in the coconut milk and broth. Add the reserved seeds, turmeric, and tamarind paste. Let it cook for 15 minutes in the preheated Air Fryer.

5. Divide between individual bowls; drizzle fresh lime juice over the top and serve immediately.

164.Grandma's Famous Pork Chops

Servings:4
Cooking Time:1 Hour 12 Minutes
Ingredients:

- 3 eggs, well-beaten
- 1 ½ cup crushed butter crackers
- 2 teaspoons mustard powder
- 1 ½ tablespoons olive oil
- 1/2 tablespoon soy sauce
- 2 tablespoons Worcestershire sauce
- ½ teaspoon dried rosemary
- 4 large-sized pork chops
- ½ teaspoon dried thyme
- 2 teaspoons fennel seeds
- Salt and freshly cracked black pepper, to taste
- 1 teaspoon red pepper flakes, crushed

Directions:

1. Add the pork chops along with olive oil, soy sauce, Worcestershire sauce, and seasonings to a resealable plastic bag. Allow pork chops to marinate for 50 minutes in your refrigerator.

2. Next step, dip the pork chops into the beaten eggs; then, coat the pork chops with the butter crackers on both sides.

3. Cook in the air fryer for 18 minutes at 405 degrees F, turning once. Bon appétit!

165.Great Pork Chops

Servings: 4
Cooking Time: 20 Minutes
Ingredients:

- 4 pork chops
- 2 tablespoons olive oil
- 2 tablespoons white flour
- 1 yellow onion, minced
- 2 garlic cloves, minced
- 2 tablespoons tomato paste
- 1 teaspoon oregano, dried
- 4 ounces red wine
- Salt and black pepper to taste

Directions:

1. In a bowl, mix the pork chops with the flour, salt, and pepper; coat the chops well.

2. Heat up the oil in a pan that fits your air fryer over medium heat.

3. Add the pork chops and brown for 2-3 minutes.

4. Add the onions, garlic, oregano, and wine; stir and cook for 2 more minutes.

5. Add the tomato paste, toss, and then place the pan into the fryer.

6. Cook at 380 degrees F for 14 minutes, and then divide between plates.

7. Serve with a side salad, and enjoy!

166.Leftover Beef And Kale Omelet

Servings:4
Cooking Time:20 Minutes
Ingredients:

- Non-stick cooking spray
- 1/2 pound leftover beef, coarsely chopped
- 2 garlic cloves, pressed
- 1 cup kale, torn into pieces and wilted
- 1 tomato, chopped
- 1/4 teaspoon brown sugar

- 4 eggs, beaten
- 4 tablespoons heavy cream
- 1/2 teaspoon turmeric powder
- Salt and ground black pepper, to your liking
- 1/8 teaspoon ground allspice

Directions:

1. Spritz the inside of four ramekins with a cooking spray.
2. Divide all of the above ingredients among the prepared ramekins. Stir until everything is well combined.
3. Air-fry at 360 degrees F for 16 minutes; check with a wooden stick and return the eggs to the Air Fryer for a few more minutes as needed. Serve immediately.

167.Ground Beef On Deep Dish Pizza

Servings:4
Cooking Time: 25 Minutes
Ingredients:

- 1 can (10-3/4 ounces) condensed tomato soup, undiluted
- 1 can (8 ounces) mushroom stems and pieces, drained
- 1 cup shredded part-skim mozzarella cheese
- 1 cup warm water (110°F to 115°F)
- 1 package (1/4 ounce) active dry yeast
- 1 small green pepper, julienned
- 1 teaspoon dried rosemary, crushed
- 1 teaspoon each dried basil, oregano and thyme
- 1 teaspoon salt
- 1 teaspoon sugar
- 1/4 teaspoon garlic powder
- 1-pound ground beef, cooked and drained
- 2 tablespoons canola oil

- 2-1/2 cups all-purpose flour

Directions:

1. In a large bowl, dissolve yeast in warm water. Add the sugar, salt, oil and 2 cups flour. Beat until smooth. Stir in enough remaining flour to form a soft dough. Cover and let rest for 20 minutes. Divide into two and store half in the freezer for future use.
2. On a floured surface, roll into a square the size of your air fryer. Transfer to a greased air fryer baking pan. Sprinkle with beef.
3. Mix well seasonings and soup in a small bowl and pour over beef.
4. Sprinkle top with mushrooms and green pepper. Top with cheese.
5. Cover pan with foil.
6. For 15 minutes, cook on 390°F.
7. Remove foil, cook for another 10 minutes or until cheese is melted.
8. Serve and enjoy.

168.Roasted Lamb

Servings:4
Cooking Time:1 Hour 30 Minutes
Ingredients:

- 2½ pounds half lamb leg roast, slits carved
- 2 garlic cloves, sliced into smaller slithers
- 1 tablespoon dried rosemary
- 1 tablespoon olive oil
- Cracked Himalayan rock salt and cracked peppercorns, to taste

Directions:

1. Preheat the Air fryer to 400 °F and grease an Air fryer basket.
2. Insert the garlic slithers in the slits and brush with rosemary, oil, salt, and black pepper.

3. Arrange the lamb in the Air fryer basket and cook for about 15 minutes.
4. Set the Air fryer to 350 °F on the Roast mode and cook for 1 hour and 15 minutes.
5. Dish out the lamb chops and serve hot.

169.Pork Tenderloin With Bacon & Veggies

Servings:3
Cooking Time: 28 Minutes
Ingredients:
- 3 potatoes
- ¾ pound frozen green beans
- 6 bacon slices
- 3 (6-ounces) pork tenderloins
- 2 tablespoons olive oil

Directions:
1. Set the temperature of air fryer to 390 degrees F. Grease an air fryer basket.
2. With a fork, pierce the potatoes.
3. Place potatoes into the prepared air fryer basket and air fry for about 15 minutes.
4. Wrap one bacon slice around 4-6 green beans.
5. Coat the pork tenderloins with oil
6. After 15 minutes, add the pork tenderloins into air fryer basket with potatoes and air fry for about 5-6 minutes.
7. Remove the pork tenderloins from basket.
8. Place bean rolls into the basket and top with the pork tenderloins.
9. Air fry for another 7 minutes.
10. Remove from air fryer and transfer the pork tenderloins onto a platter.
11. Cut each tenderloin into desired size slices.

12. Serve alongside the potatoes and green beans rolls.

170.Bacon-cheeseburger Casserole

Servings:6
Cooking Time: 35 Minutes
Ingredients:
- 1 small onion, chopped
- 1 tablespoon ground mustard
- 1 tablespoon Worcestershire sauce
- 1/2 can (15 ounces) tomato sauce
- 1/2 cup grape tomatoes, chopped
- 1/2 cup shredded cheddar cheese
- 1/4 cup sliced dill pickles
- 1-pound ground beef
- 4-ounces process cheese (Velveeta)
- 6 bacon strips, cooked and crumbled
- 8-ounces frozen Tater Tots

Directions:
1. Lightly grease baking pan of air fryer with cooking spray. Add beef and half of onions.
2. For 10 minutes, cook on 390°F. Halfway through cooking time, stir and crumble beef.
3. Stir in Worcestershire, mustard, Velveeta, and tomato sauce. Mix well. Cook for 4 minutes until melted.
4. Mix well and evenly spread in pan. Top with cheddar cheese and then bacon strips.
5. Evenly top with tater tots. Cover pan with foil.
6. Cook for 15 minutes at 390°F. Uncover and bake for 10 minutes more until tops are lightly browned.
7. Serve and enjoy topped with pickles and tomatoes and remaining onion.

171.Easy & The Traditional Beef Roast Recipe

Servings:12

Cooking Time: 2 Hours

Ingredients:

- 1 cup organic beef broth
- 3 pounds beef round roast
- 4 tablespoons olive oil
- Salt and pepper to taste

Directions:

1. Place in a Ziploc bag all the ingredients and allow to marinate in the fridge for 2 hours.
2. Preheat the air fryer for 5 minutes.
3. Transfer all ingredients in a baking dish that will fit in the air fryer.
4. Place in the air fryer and cook for 2 hours for 400 °F.

172.Mouthwatering Pork Medallions With Creole Mustard

Servings: 4

Cooking Time: 25 Minutes

Ingredients:

- 1 pound pork medallions, trimmed and sliced into thick medallions
- 2 tablespoons Creole mustard
- ½ tablespoon apple cider vinegar
- 1 ½ tablespoons extra-virgin olive oil
- 2 teaspoon cumin seeds, ground
- ½ teaspoon seasoned salt
- 1/3 teaspoon freshly cracked black peppercorns, or multi-color peppercorns

Directions:

1. Toss the pork medallions with all the other items until well coated. Cook in your Air Fryer for 13 minutes at 365 degrees F.
2. Check for doneness and cook for 4 to 5 minutes longer as needed.
3. To finish, mound the wilted kale onto a serving plate. Top with the beef medallions and serve immediately.

173.Salami Rolls With Homemade Mustard Spread

Servings:4

Cooking Time:10 Minutes

Ingredients:

- 7 ounces Manchego cheese, grated
- 2/3 pound pork salami, chopped
- 7 ounces canned crescent rolls
- For the Mustard Spread:
- 1 tablespoon sour cream
- 1/3 teaspoon garlic powder
- 1/3 cup mayonnaise
- 2 ½ tablespoons spicy brown mustard
- Salt, to taste

Directions:

1. Start by preheating your air fryer to 325 degrees F. Now, form the crescent rolls into "sheets".
2. Place the chopped Manchego and pork salami in the middle of each dough sheet.
3. Shape the dough into the rolls; bake the rolls for 8 minutes. Then, decrease the temperature and bake at 290 degrees F for 5 more minutes.
4. In the meantime, combine all of the ingredients for the mustard spread. Arrange the warm rolls on a serving platter and serve with the mustard spread on the side. Enjoy!

174.Lamb And Salsa

Servings: 4

Cooking Time: 35 Minutes

Ingredients:

- 1 tablespoon chipotle powder
- A pinch of salt and black pepper
- 1 and ½ pounds lamb loin, cubed
- 2 tablespoons red vinegar
- 4 tablespoons olive oil

- 2 tomatoes, cubed
- 2 cucumbers, sliced
- 2 spring onions, chopped
- Juice of ½ lemon
- ¼ cup mint, chopped

Directions:

1. Heat up a pan that fits your air fryer with half of the oil over medium-high heat, add the lamb, stir and brown for 5 minutes. Add the chipotle powder, salt pepper and the vinegar, toss, put the pan in the air fryer and cook at 380 degrees F for 30 minutes. In a bowl, mix tomatoes with cucumbers, onions, lemon juice, mint and the rest of the oil and toss. Divide the lamb between plates, top each serving with the cucumber salsa and serve.

175.Ground Beef, Rice'n Cabbage Casserole

Servings:6
Cooking Time: 50 Minutes
Ingredients:

- 1-pound ground beef
- 1 (14 ounce) can beef broth
- 1/2 cup chopped onion
- 1/2 (29 ounce) can tomato sauce
- 1/2 cup uncooked white rice
- 1/2 teaspoon salt
- 1-3/4 pounds chopped cabbage

Directions:

1. Lightly grease baking pan of air fryer with cooking spray. Add beef and for 10 minutes, cook on 360°F. Halfway through cooking time, stir and crumble beef.
2. Meanwhile, in a large bowl whisk well salt, rice, cabbage, onion, and tomato sauce. Add to pan of meat and mix well. Pour broth.

3. Cover pan with foil.
4. Cook for 25 minutes at 330°F, uncover, mix and cook for another 15 minutes.
5. Serve and enjoy.

176.Beef With Ghee Mushroom Mix

Servings: 4
Cooking Time: 25 Minutes
Ingredients:

- 4 beef steaks
- 1 tablespoon olive oil
- A pinch of salt and black pepper
- 2 tablespoons ghee, melted
- 2 garlic cloves, minced
- 5 cups wild mushrooms, sliced
- 1 tablespoon parsley, chopped

Directions:

1. Heat up a pan that fits the air fryer with the oil over medium-high heat, add the steaks and sear them for 2 minutes on each side. Add the rest of the ingredients, toss, transfer the pan to your air fryer and cook at 380 degrees F for 20 minutes. Divide between plates and serve.

177.Garlic Dill Leg Of Lamb

Servings: 2
Cooking Time: 21 Minutes
Ingredients:

- 9 oz leg of lamb, boneless
- 1 teaspoon minced garlic
- 2 tablespoons butter, softened
- ½ teaspoon dried dill
- ½ teaspoon salt

Directions:

1. In the shallow bowl mix up minced garlic, butter, dried dill, and salt. Then rub the leg of lamb with butter mixture and place it in the air fryer. Cook it at 380F for 21 minutes.

178.Basil Beef And Avocado

Servings: 4
Cooking Time: 25 Minutes
Ingredients:

- 4 flank steaks
- 1 garlic clove, minced
- 1/3 cup beef stock
- 2 avocados, peeled, pitted and sliced
- 1 teaspoon chili flakes
- ½ cup basil, chopped
- 2 spring onions, chopped
- 2 teaspoons olive oil
- A pinch of salt and black pepper

Directions:

1. Heat up a pan that fits the air fryer with the oil over medium-high heat, add the steaks and cook for 2 minutes on each side. Add the rest of the ingredients except the avocados, put the pan in the air fryer and cook at 380 degrees F for 15 minutes. Add the avocado slices, cook for 5 minutes more, divide everything between plates and serve.

179.Moroccan Beef Kebab

Servings: 4
Cooking Time: 30 Minutes
Ingredients:

- 1/2 cup leeks, chopped
- 2 garlic cloves, smashed
- 2 pounds ground chuck
- Salt, to taste
- 1/4 teaspoon ground black pepper, or more to taste
- 1 teaspoon cayenne pepper
- 1/2 teaspoon ground sumac
- 3 saffron threads
- 2 tablespoons loosely packed fresh continental parsley leaves
- 4 tablespoons tahini sauce
- 4 ounces baby arugula
- 1 tomato, cut into slices

Directions:

1. In a bowl, mix the chopped leeks, garlic, ground chuck, and spices; knead with your hands until everything is well incorporated.
2. Now, mound the beef mixture around a wooden skewer into a pointed-ended sausage.
3. Cook in the preheated Air Fryer at 360 degrees F for 25 minutes.
4. Serve your kebab with the tahini sauce baby arugula and tomato. Enjoy!

180.Rosemary Lamb Steak

Servings: 2
Cooking Time: 12 Minutes
Ingredients:

- 12 oz lamb steak (6 oz each lamb steak)
- 1 teaspoon dried rosemary
- 1 teaspoon minced onion
- 1 tablespoon avocado oil
- ½ teaspoon salt

Directions:

1. Rub the lamb steaks with minced onion and salt. In the shallow bowl mix up dried rosemary and avocado oil. Sprinkle the meat with rosemary mixture. After this, preheat the air fryer to 400F. Put the lamb steaks in the air fryer in one layer and cook them for 6 minutes. Then flip the meat on another side and cook it for 6 minutes more.

181.Fried Sausage And Mushrooms Recipe

Servings: 6
Cooking Time:50 Minutes
Ingredients:

- 3 red bell peppers; chopped
- 2 sweet onions; chopped.
- 1 tbsp. brown sugar
- 1 tsp. olive oil
- 2 lbs. pork sausage; sliced
- Salt and black pepper to the taste
- 2 lbs. Portobello mushrooms; sliced

Directions:

1. In a baking dish that fits your air fryer, mix sausage slices with oil, salt, pepper, bell pepper, mushrooms, onion and sugar, toss, introduce in your air fryer and cook at 300 °F, for 40 minutes. Divide among plates and serve right away.

182. Nana's Pork Chops With Cilantro

Servings: 6
Cooking Time: 22 Minutes
Ingredients:
- 1/3 cup pork rinds
- Roughly chopped fresh cilantro, to taste
- 2 teaspoons Cajun seasonings
- Nonstick cooking spray
- 2 eggs, beaten
- 3 tablespoons almond meal
- 1 teaspoon seasoned salt
- Garlic & onion spice blend, to taste
- 6 pork chops
- 1/3 teaspoon freshly cracked black pepper

Directions:
1. Coat the pork chops with Cajun seasonings, salt, pepper, and the spice blend on all sides.
2. Then, add the almond meal to a plate. In a shallow dish, whisk the egg until pale and smooth. Place the pork rinds in the third bowl.
3. Dredge each pork piece in the almond meal; then, coat them with the egg; finally, coat them with the pork rinds. Spritz them with cooking spray on both sides.
4. Now, air-fry pork chops for about 18 minutes at 345 degrees F; make sure to taste for doneness after first 12 minutes of cooking. Lastly, garnish with fresh cilantro. Bon appétit!

183. Pickling 'n Jerk Spiced Pork

Servings: 3
Cooking Time: 15 Minutes

Ingredients:
- ½ cup ready-made jerk sauce
- 1 cup rum
- 1 cup water
- 1-lb pork tenderloin, sliced into 1-inch cubes
- 2 teaspoons pickling spices
- 3 tablespoons brown sugar
- 3 tablespoons each salt
- 4 garlic cloves

Directions:
1. In a saucepan, bring to a boil water salt and brown sugar. Stir in garlic and pickling spices and simmer for 3 minutes. Turn off fire and whisk in rum.
2. Transfer sauce to a shallow dish, mix well pork tenderloin and marinate in the ref for 3 hours.
3. Thread pork pieces in skewers. Baste with jerk sauce and place on skewer rack in air fryer.
4. For 12 minutes, cook on 360°F. Halfway through cooking time, turnover skewers and baste with sauce. If needed, cook in batches.
5. Serve and enjoy.

184. Pork Butt With Herb-garlic Sauce

Servings: 4
Cooking Time: 35 Minutes + Marinating Time
Ingredients:
- 1 pound pork butt, cut into pieces 2-inches long
- 1 teaspoon golden flaxseed meal
- 1 egg white, well whisked
- Salt and ground black pepper, to taste
- 1 tablespoon olive oil
- 1 tablespoon coconut aminos
- 1 teaspoon lemon juice, preferably freshly squeezed
- For the Coriander-Garlic Sauce:
- 3 garlic cloves, peeled
- 1/3 cup fresh parsley leaves
- 1/3 cup fresh coriander leaves
- 1/2 tablespoon salt

- 1 teaspoon lemon juice
- 1/3 cup extra-virgin olive oil

Directions:
1. Combine the pork strips with the flaxseed meal, egg white, salt, pepper, olive oil, coconut aminos, and lemon juice. Cover and refrigerate for 30 to 45 minutes.
2. After that, spritz the pork strips with a nonstick cooking spray.
3. Set your Air Fryer to cook at 380 degrees F. Press the power button and air-fry for 15 minutes; pause the machine, shake the basket and cook for 15 more minutes.
4. Meanwhile, puree the garlic in a food processor until finely minced. Now, puree the parsley, coriander, salt, and lemon juice. With the machine running, carefully pour in the olive oil.
5. Serve the pork with well-chilled sauce with and enjoy!

185.Honey Mustard Cheesy Meatballs

Servings:8
Cooking Time:15 Minutes
Ingredients:
- 2 onions, chopped
- 1 pound ground beef
- 4 tablespoons fresh basil, chopped
- 2 tablespoons cheddar cheese, grated
- 2 teaspoons garlic paste
- 2 teaspoons honey
- Salt and black pepper, to taste
- 2 teaspoons mustard

Directions:

1. Preheat the Air fryer to 385 °F and grease an Air fryer basket.
2. Mix all the ingredients in a bowl until well combined.
3. Shape the mixture into equal-sized balls gently and arrange the meatballs in the Air fryer basket.
4. Cook for about 15 minutes and dish out to serve warm.

186.Meatballs'n Parmesan-cheddar Pizza

Servings:4
Cooking Time: 15 Minutes
Ingredients:
- 1 prebaked 6-inch pizza crust
- 1 teaspoon garlic powder
- 1 teaspoon Italian seasoning
- 4 tbsp grated Parmesan cheese
- 1 small onion, halved and sliced
- 1/2 can (8 ounces) pizza sauce
- 6 frozen fully cooked Italian meatballs (1/2 ounce each), thawed and halved
- 1/2 cup shredded part-skim mozzarella cheese
- 1/2 cup shredded cheddar cheese

Directions:
1. Lightly grease baking pan of air fryer with cooking spray.
2. Place crust on bottom of pan. Spread sauce on top. Sprinkle with parmesan, Italian seasoning, and garlic powder.
3. Top with meatballs and onion. Sprinkle remaining cheese.
4. For 15 minutes, cook on preheated 390°F air fryer.
5. Serve and enjoy.

FISH & SEAFOOD RECIPES

187.Jamaican-style Fish And Potato Fritters

Servings: 2
Cooking Time: 30 Minutes
Ingredients:
- 1/2 pound sole fillets
- 1/2 pound mashed potatoes
- 1 egg, well beaten
- 1/2 cup red onion, chopped
- 2 garlic cloves, minced
- 2 tablespoons fresh parsley, chopped
- 1 bell pepper, finely chopped
- 1/2 teaspoon scotch bonnet pepper, minced
- 1 tablespoon olive oil
- 1 tablespoon coconut aminos
- 1/2 teaspoon paprika
- Salt and white pepper, to taste

Directions:
1. Start by preheating your Air Fryer to 395 degrees F. Spritz the sides and bottom of the cooking basket with cooking spray.
2. Cook the sole fillets in the preheated Air Fryer for 10 minutes, flipping them halfway through the cooking time.
3. In a mixing bowl, mash the sole fillets into flakes. Stir in the remaining ingredients. Shape the fish mixture into patties.
4. Bake in the preheated Air Fryer at 390 degrees F for 14 minutes, flipping them halfway through the cooking time. Bon appétit!

188.Shrimp And Celery Salad

Servings: 4
Cooking Time: 5 Minutes

Ingredients:
- 3 oz chevre
- 1 teaspoon avocado oil
- ½ teaspoon dried oregano
- 8 oz shrimps, peeled
- 1 teaspoon butter, melted
- ½ teaspoon salt
- ½ teaspoon chili flakes
- 4 oz celery stalk, chopped

Directions:
1. Sprinkle the shrimps with dried oregano and melted butter and put in the air fryer. Cook the seafood at 400F for 5 minutes. Meanwhile, crumble the chevre. Put the chopped celery stalk in the salad bowl. Add crumbled chevre, chili flakes, salt, and avocado oil. Mix up the salad well and top it with cooked shrimps.

189.Salted Tequila 'n Lime Shrimp

Servings:3
Cooking Time: 16 Minutes
Ingredients:
- 1 large lime, quartered
- 1 pinch garlic salt
- 1 pinch ground cumin
- 1/4 cup olive oil
- 1-pound large shrimp, peeled and deveined
- 2 tablespoons lime juice
- 2 tablespoons tequila
- ground black pepper to taste

Directions:
1. In a bowl mix well pepper, cumin, salt, olive oil, tequila and lime juice. Stir in shrimp and marinate for at least an hour. Tossing every now and then.

2. Thread shrimps in skewers. Place on skewer rack. If needed cook in batches.
3. For 8 minutes, cook on 360°F. Halfway through cooking time,
4. Serve and enjoy.

190.Fried Shrimp With Chipotle Sauce

Servings: 4
Cooking Time: 10 Minutes
Ingredients:
- 12 jumbo shrimp
- 1/2 teaspoon garlic salt
- 1/4 teaspoon freshly cracked mixed peppercorns
- For the Sauce:
- 1 teaspoon Dijon mustard
- 4 tablespoons mayonnaise
- 1 teaspoon lemon rind, grated
- 1 teaspoon chipotle powder
- 1/2 teaspoon cumin powder

Directions:
1. Season your shrimp with garlic salt and cracked peppercorns.
2. Now, air-fry them in the cooking basket at 395 degrees F for 5 minutes. After that, pause the machine. Flip them over and set the timer for 2 more minutes.
3. Meanwhile, mix all ingredients for the sauce; whisk to combine well. Serve with the warm shrimps. Bon appétit!

191.Another Crispy Coconut Shrimp Recipe

Servings:4
Cooking Time: 20 Minutes
Ingredients:
- ½ cup flour
- ½ stick cold butter, cut into cubes
- ½ tablespoon lemon juice
- 1 egg yolk, beaten

- 1 green onion, chopped
- 1-pound salmon fillets, cut into small cubes
- 3 tablespoons whipping cream
- 4 eggs, beaten
- Salt and pepper to taste

Directions:
1. Preheat the air fryer to 390 °F.
2. Season salmon fillets with lemon juice, salt and pepper.
3. In another bowl, combine the flour and butter. Add cold water gradually to form a dough. Knead the dough on a flat surface to form a sheet.
4. Place the dough on the baking dish and press firmly on the dish.
5. Beat the eggs and egg yolk and season with salt and pepper to taste.
6. Place the salmon cubes on the pan lined with dough and pour the egg over.
7. Cook for 15 to 20 minutes.
8. Garnish with green onions once cooked.

192.Red Hot Chili Fish Curry

Servings: 4
Cooking Time: 25 Minutes
Ingredients:
- 2 tablespoons sunflower oil
- 1 pound fish, chopped
- 2 red chilies, chopped
- 1 tablespoon coriander powder
- 1 teaspoon red curry paste
- 1 cup coconut milk
- Salt and white pepper, to taste
- 1/2 teaspoon fenugreek seeds
- 1 shallot, minced
- 1 garlic clove, minced
- 1 ripe tomato, pureed

Directions:

1. Preheat your Air Fryer to 380 degrees F; brush the cooking basket with 1 tablespoon of sunflower oil.
2. Cook your fish for 10 minutes on both sides. Transfer to the baking pan that is previously greased with the remaining tablespoon of sunflower oil.
3. Add the remaining ingredients and reduce the heat to 350 degrees F. Continue to cook an additional 10 to 12 minutes or until everything is heated through. Enjoy!

193.Sweet Honey-hoisin Glazed Salmon

Servings:2
Cooking Time: 12 Minutes
Ingredients:

- 1 tablespoon honey
- 1 tablespoon olive oil
- 1 tablespoon rice wine
- 1 tablespoon soy sauce
- 1-lb salmon filet, cut into 2-inch rectangles
- 3 tablespoons hoisin sauce

Directions:
1. In a shallow dish, mix well all Ingredients. Marinate in the ref for 3 hours.
2. Thread salmon pieces in skewers and reserve marinade for basting. Place on skewer rack in air fryer.
3. For 12 minutes, cook on 360°F. Halfway through cooking time, turnover skewers and baste with marinade. If needed, cook in batches.
4. Serve and enjoy.

194.Rich Crab Croquettes

Servings:4
Cooking Time: 30 Minutes
Ingredients:

- 1 ½ lb lump crab meat
- 3 egg whites, beaten
- ⅓ cup sour cream
- ⅓ cup mayonnaise
- 1 ½ tbsp olive oil
- 1 red pepper, chopped finely
- ⅓ cup chopped red onion
- 2 ½ tbsp chopped celery
- ½ tsp chopped tarragon
- ½ tsp chopped chives
- 1 tsp chopped parsley
- 1 tsp cayenne pepper
- Breading:
- 1 ½ cup breadcrumbs
- 2 tsp olive oil
- 1 cup flour
- 4 eggs, beaten
- Salt to taste

Directions:
1. Place a skillet over medium heat on a stovetop, add 1 ½ tbsp olive oil, red pepper, onion, and celery. Sauté for 5 minutes or until sweaty and translucent. Turn off heat. Add the breadcrumbs, the remaining olive oil, and salt to a food processor. Blend to mix evenly; set aside. In 2 separate bowls, add the flour and 4 eggs respectively, set aside.
2. In a separate bowl, add crabmeat, mayo, egg whites, sour cream, tarragon, chives, parsley, cayenne pepper, and celery sauté and mix evenly. Form bite-sized balls from the mixture and place onto a plate.
3. Preheat the air fryer to 390 F. Dip each crab meatball (croquettes) in the egg mixture and press them in the breadcrumb mixture. Place the croquettes in the fryer basket, avoid overcrowding. Close the air fryer and

cook for 10 minutes or until golden brown. Remove them and plate them. Serve the crab croquettes with tomato dipping sauce and a side of vegetable fries.

195.Grilled Shrimp With Butter

Servings:4
Cooking Time: 15 Minutes
Ingredients:

- 6 tablespoons unsalted butter
- ½ cup red onion, chopped
- 1 ½ teaspoon red pepper
- 1 teaspoon shrimp paste or fish sauce
- 1 ½ teaspoon lime juice
- Salt and pepper to taste
- 24 large shrimps, shelled and deveined

Directions:

1. Preheat the air fryer at 390 °F.
2. Place the grill pan accessory in the air fryer.
3. Place all ingredients in a Ziploc bag and give a good shake.
4. Skewer the shrimps through a bamboo skewer and place on the grill pan.
5. Cook for 15 minutes.
6. Flip the shrimps halfway through the cooking time.

196.Shrimp With Garlic And Goat Cheese

Servings: 2
Cooking Time: 10 Minutes
Ingredients:

- 1/2 tablespoon fresh parsley, roughly chopped
- 1 ½ tablespoons balsamic vinegar
- Sea salt flakes, to taste
- 1 pound shrimp, deveined
- 1 tablespoon coconut aminos
- 1 teaspoon Dijon mustard
- 1/2 teaspoon garlic powder
- 1 ½ tablespoons olive oil
- 1/2 teaspoon smoked cayenne pepper
- Salt and ground black peppercorns, to savor
- 1 cup goat cheese, shredded

Directions:

1. Set the Air Fryer to cook at 385 degrees F.
2. In a bowl, thoroughly combine all ingredients, except for cheese.
3. Dump the shrimp into the cooking basket; air-fry for 7 to 8 minutes. Bon appétit!

197.Tuna Au Gratin With Herbs

Servings: 4
Cooking Time: 20 Minutes
Ingredients:

- 1 tablespoon butter, melted
- 1 medium-sized leek, thinly sliced
- 1 tablespoon chicken stock
- 1 tablespoon dry white wine
- 1 pound tuna
- 1/2 teaspoon red pepper flakes, crushed
- Sea salt and ground black pepper, to taste
- 1/2 teaspoon dried rosemary
- 1/2 teaspoon dried basil
- 1/2 teaspoon dried thyme
- 2 small ripe tomatoes, pureed
- 1 cup Parmesan cheese, grated

Directions:

1. Melt 1/2 tablespoon of butter in a sauté pan over medium-high heat. Now, cook the leek and garlic until tender and aromatic. Add the stock and wine to deglaze the pan.

2. Preheat your Air Fryer to 370 degrees F.
3. Grease a casserole dish with the remaining 1/2 tablespoon of melted butter. Place the fish in the casserole dish. Add the seasonings. Top with the sautéed leek mixture.
4. Add the tomato puree. Cook for 10 minutes in the preheated Air Fryer. Top with grated Parmesan cheese; cook an additional 7 minutes until the crumbs are golden. Bon appétit!

198.Coriander Cod And Green Beans

Servings: 4
Cooking Time: 15 Minutes
Ingredients:
- 12 oz cod fillet
- ½ cup green beans, trimmed and halved
- 1 tablespoon avocado oil
- 1 teaspoon salt
- 1 teaspoon ground coriander

Directions:
1. Cut the cod fillet on 4 servings and sprinkle every serving with salt and ground coriander. After this, place the fish on 4 foil squares. Top them with green beans and avocado oil and wrap them into parcels. Preheat the air fryer to 400F. Place the cod parcels in the air fryer and cook them for 15 minutes.

199.Fried Haddock Fillets

Servings: 2
Cooking Time: 20 Minutes
Ingredients:
- 2 haddock fillets
- 1/2 cup parmesan cheese, freshly grated
- 1 teaspoon dried parsley flakes
- 1 egg, beaten
- 1/2 teaspoon coarse sea salt
- 1/4 teaspoon ground black pepper
- 1/4 teaspoon cayenne pepper
- 2 tablespoons olive oil

Directions:
1. Start by preheating your Air Fryer to 360 degrees F. Pat dry the haddock fillets and set aside.
2. In a shallow bowl, thoroughly combine the parmesan and parsley flakes. Mix until everything is well incorporated.
3. In a separate shallow bowl, whisk the egg with salt, black pepper, and cayenne pepper.
4. Dip the haddock fillets into the egg. Then, dip the fillets into the parmesan mixture until well coated on all sides.
5. Drizzle the olive oil all over the fish fillets. Lower the coated fillets into the lightly greased Air Fryer basket. Cook for 11 to 13 minutes. Bon appétit!

200.Basil Paprika Calamari

Servings: 2
Cooking Time: 4 Minutes
Ingredients:
- 8 oz calamari, peeled, trimmed
- 1 teaspoon ghee, melted
- 1 teaspoon fresh basil, chopped
- ½ teaspoon smoked paprika
- ½ teaspoon white pepper
- 1 tablespoon apple cider vinegar

Directions:
1. In the shallow bowl mix up melted ghee, basil, smoked paprika, white pepper, and apple cider vinegar. After this, sprinkle the calamari with ghee

mixture and leave for 15 minutes to marinate. After this, roughly slice the calamari. Preheat the air fryer to 400F. Put the sliced calamari in the air fryer and cook for 2 minutes. Shake the seafood well and cook for 2 minutes more.

201. Thyme Scallops

Servings: 1
Cooking Time: 12 Minutes
Ingredients:
- 1 lb. scallops
- Salt and pepper
- ½ tbsp. butter
- ½ cup thyme, chopped

Directions:
1. Wash the scallops and dry them completely. Season with pepper and salt, then set aside while you prepare the pan.
2. Grease a foil pan in several spots with the butter and cover the bottom with the thyme. Place the scallops on top.
3. Pre-heat the fryer at 400°F and set the rack inside.
4. Place the foil pan on the rack and allow to cook for seven minutes.
5. Take care when removing the pan from the fryer and transfer the scallops to a serving dish. Spoon any remaining butter in the pan over the fish and enjoy.

202. Grilled Squid Rings With Kale And Tomatoes

Servings: 3
Cooking Time: 15 Minutes
Ingredients:
- 1 2-pound squid, cleaned and sliced into rings
- Salt and pepper to taste
- 3 cloves of garlic, minced
- 1 sprig rosemary, chopped
- ¼ cup red wine vinegar
- 3 pounds kale, torn
- 3 tomatoes, chopped

Directions:
1. Preheat the air fryer at 390 °F.
2. Place the grill pan accessory in the air fryer.
3. Season the squid rings with salt, pepper, garlic, rosemary, and wine vinegar.
4. Grill for 15 minutes.
5. Serve octopus on a bed of kale leaves and garnish with tomatoes on top.

203. Tuna Steaks With Pearl Onions

Servings: 4
Cooking Time: 20 Minutes
Ingredients:
- 4 tuna steaks
- 1 pound pearl onions
- 4 teaspoons olive oil
- 1 teaspoon dried rosemary
- 1 teaspoon dried marjoram
- 1 tablespoon cayenne pepper
- 1/2 teaspoon sea salt
- 1/2 teaspoon black pepper, preferably freshly cracked
- 1 lemon, sliced

Directions:
1. Place the tuna steaks in the lightly greased cooking basket. Top with the pearl onions; add the olive oil, rosemary, marjoram, cayenne pepper, salt, and black pepper.
2. Bake in the preheated Air Fryer at 400 degrees F for 9 to 10 minutes. Work in two batches.
3. Serve warm with lemon slices and enjoy!

204. Air Fried Calamari

Servings: 3
Cooking Time: 30 Minutes
Ingredients:
- ½ cup cornmeal or cornstarch

- 2 large eggs, beaten
- 2 mashed garlic cloves
- 1 cup breadcrumbs
- lemon juice

Directions:

1. Coat calamari with the cornmeal. The first mixture is prepared by mixing the eggs and garlic. Dip the calamari in the eggs' mixture. Then dip them in the breadcrumbs. Put the rings in the fridge for 2 hours.
2. Then, line them in the air fryer and add oil generously. Fry for 10 to 13 minutes at 390 F, shaking once halfway through. Serve with garlic mayonnaise and top with lemon juice.

205.Creole Crab

Servings: 6
Cooking Time: 6 Minutes
Ingredients:

- 1 teaspoon Creole seasonings
- 4 tablespoons almond flour
- ¼ teaspoon baking powder
- 1 teaspoon apple cider vinegar
- ¼ teaspoon onion powder
- 1 teaspoon dried dill
- 1 teaspoon ghee
- 13 oz crab meat, finely chopped
- 1 egg, beaten
- Cooking spray

Directions:

1. In the mixing bowl mix up crab meat, egg, dried dill, ghee, onion powder, apple cider vinegar, baking powder, and Creole seasonings. Then add almond flour and stir the mixture with the help of the fork until it is homogenous. Make the small balls (hushpuppies). Preheat the air fryer to 390F. Put the hushpuppies in the air fryer basket and spray with cooking spray. Cook them for 3 minutes. Then flip them on another side and cook for 3 minutes more or

until the hushpuppies are golden brown.

206.Old Bay 'n Dijon Seasoned Crab Cakes

Servings:2
Cooking Time: 10 Minutes
Ingredients:

- ¼ cup chopped green onion
- ½ cup panko
- 1 ½ teaspoon old bay seasoning
- 1 teaspoon Dijon mustard
- 1 teaspoon Worcestershire sauce
- 1-pound lump crab meat
- 2 large eggs
- Salt and pepper to taste

Directions:

1. Preheat the air fryer to 390 °F.
2. Place the grill pan accessory in the air fryer.
3. In a mixing bowl, combine all Ingredients until everything is well-incorporated.
4. Use your hands to form small patties of crab cakes.
5. Place on the grill pan and cook for 10 minutes.
6. Flip the crab cakes halfway through the cooking time for even browning.

207.Tasty Sockeye Fish

Servings:2
Cooking Time: 25 Minutes
Ingredients:

- ½ bulb fennel, thinly sliced
- 4 tbsp melted butter
- Salt and pepper to taste
- 1-2 tsp fresh dill
- 2 sockeye salmon fillets
- 8 cherry tomatoes, halved
- ¼ cup fish stock

Directions:

1. Preheat air fryer to 400 F. Bring to a boil salted water over medium heat. Add the potatoes and blanch for 2 minutes; drain. Cut 2 large-sized

rectangles of parchment paper of 13x15 inch size.

2. In a large bowl, mix potatoes, fennel, pepper, and salt. Divide the mixture between parchment paper pieces and sprinkle with dill. Top with fillets. Add cherry tomatoes on top and drizzle with butter; pour fish stock on top. Fold the squares and seal them. Cook the packets in the air fryer for 10 minutes.

208.Hot Salmon & Broccoli

Servings:2
Cooking Time: 25 Minutes
Ingredients:
- 1 tsp olive oil
- Juice of 1 lime
- 1 tsp chili flakes
- Salt and black pepper
- 1 head of broccoli, cut into florets
- 1 tsp olive oil
- 1 tbsp soy sauce

Directions:
1. In a bowl, add oil, lime juice, flakes, salt, and black pepper; rub the mixture onto fillets. Lay the florets into your air fryer and drizzle with oil. Arrange the fillets around or on top and cook at 340 F for 10 minutes. Drizzle the florets with soy sauce to serve!

209.Air Fried Catfish

Servings: 4
Cooking Time: 20 Minutes
Ingredients:
- 4 catfish fillets
- 1 tbsp olive oil
- 1/4 cup fish seasoning
- 1 tbsp fresh parsley, chopped

Directions:
1. Preheat the air fryer to 400 F.
2. Spray air fryer basket with cooking spray.

3. Seasoned fish with seasoning and place into the air fryer basket.
4. Drizzle fish fillets with oil and cook for 10 minutes.
5. Turn fish to another side and cook for 10 minutes more.
6. Garnish with parsley and serve.

210.Simple Salmon Patties

Servings: 2
Cooking Time: 10 Minutes
Ingredients:
- 14 oz salmon
- 1/2 onion, diced
- 1 egg, lightly beaten
- 1 tsp dill
- 1/2 cup almond flour

Directions:
1. Spray air fryer basket with cooking spray.
2. Add all ingredients into the bowl and mix until well combined.
3. Spray air fryer basket with cooking spray.
4. Make patties from salmon mixture and place into the air fryer basket.
5. Cook at 370 F for 5 minutes.
6. Turn patties to another side and cook for 5 minutes more.
7. Serve and enjoy.

211.Japanese Ponzu Marinated Tuna

Servings:4
Cooking Time: 10 Minutes
Ingredients:
- 1 cup Japanese ponzu sauce
- 2 tbsp sesame oil
- 1 tbsp red pepper flakes
- 2 tbsp ginger paste
- ¼ cup scallions, sliced
- Salt and black pepper to taste

Directions:
1. In a bowl, mix the ponzu sauce, sesame oil, red pepper flakes, ginger paste, salt, and black pepper. Add in the tuna and toss to coat. Cover and

leave to marinate for 60 minutes in the fridge.

2. Preheat air Fryer to 380 F. Spray air fryer basket with cooking spray. Remove tuna from the fridge and arrange on the air fryer basket. Cook for 6 minutes, turning once. Top with scallions to serve.

212. 3-ingredients Catfish

Servings:4
Cooking Time: 23 Minutes
Ingredients:
- 4 (6-ounces) catfish fillets
- ¼ cup seasoned fish fry
- 1 tablespoon olive oil

Directions:
1. Set the temperature of air fryer to 400 degrees F. Grease an air fryer basket.
2. In a bowl, add the catfish fillets and seasoned fish fry. Toss to coat well.
3. Then, drizzle each fillet evenly with oil.
4. Arrange catfish fillets into the prepared air fryer basket in a single layer.
5. Air fry for about 10 minutes.
6. Flip the side and spray with the cooking spray.
7. Air fry for another 10 minutes.
8. Flip one last time and air fry for about 2-3 more minutes.
9. Remove from air fryer and transfer the catfish fillets onto serving plates.
10. Serve hot.

213. Cajun Salmon

Servings: 1
Cooking Time: 20 Minutes
Ingredients:
- 1 salmon fillet
- Cajun seasoning
- Light sprinkle of sugar
- ¼ lemon, juiced, to serve

Directions:
1. 1 Pre-heat Air Fryer to 355°F.

2. 2 Lightly cover all sides of the salmon with Cajun seasoning. Sprinkle conservatively with sugar.
3. 3 For a salmon fillet about three-quarters of an inch thick, cook in the fryer for 7 minutes, skin-side-up on the grill pan.
4. 4 Serve with the lemon juice.

214. Turmeric Spiced Salmon With Soy Sauce

Servings:4
Cooking Time: 12 Minutes
Ingredients:
- ½ tablespoon sugar
- ½ tablespoon turmeric powder
- 1 cup cherry tomatoes
- 1 slab of salmon fillets, sliced into cubes
- 1 tablespoon soy sauce
- A dash of black pepper
- Chopped coriander for garnish

Directions:
1. Season the salmon fillets with turmeric powder, sugar, soy sauce, and black pepper. Allow to marinate for 30 minutes in the fridge.
2. Preheat the air fryer to 330 °F.
3. Skewer the salmon cubes alternating with tomatoes.
4. Place on the double layer rack.
5. Cook for 10 to 12 minutes.

215. Old Bay Crab Sticks With Garlic Mayo

Servings:4
Cooking Time: 20 Minutes
Ingredients:
- 1 tbsp old bay seasoning
- ⅓ cup panko breadcrumbs
- 1 egg
- ¼ cup mayonnaise
- 2 garlic cloves, minced
- 1 lime, juiced
- 1 tsp flour

Directions:

1. Preheat your Air Fryer to 390 F. Spray the air fryer basket with cooking spray.
2. Beat the eggs in a bowl. In a separate bowl, mix panko breadcrumbs with old bay seasoning. In a third bowl, pour the flour.
3. Dip the crab sticks in the flour and then in the eggs, and finally in the breadcrumb mixture. Spray with cooking spray and arrange on the cooking basket. Cook for 12 minutes, flipping halfway through.
4. Meanwhile, mix well all the mayonnaise with garlic and lime juice. Serve with crab sticks.

216.Grilled Barramundi In Lemon Sauce

Servings:3
Cooking Time: 25 Minutes
Ingredients:
- 2 lemons, juiced
- Salt and pepper to taste
- 6 oz butter
- ¾ cup thickened cream
- ½ cup white wine
- 2 bay leaves
- 15 black peppercorns
- 2 cloves garlic, minced
- 2 shallots, chopped

Directions:
1. Preheat the air fryer to 390 F. Place the barramundi fillets on a baking paper and put them in the fryer basket. Cook for 15 minutes. Remove to a serving platter without the paper.
2. Place a small pan over low heat on a stovetop. Add the garlic and shallots, and dry fry for 20 seconds. Add the wine, bay leaves, and peppercorns. Stir and allow the liquid to reduce by three quarters, and add the cream.

Stir and let the sauce thicken into a dark cream color.
3. Add the butter, whisk it into the cream until it has fully melted. Add the lemon juice, pepper, and salt. Strain the sauce into a serving bowl. Pour the sauce over the fish and serve with a side of rice.

217.Coconut Prawns

Servings: 4
Cooking Time: 10 Minutes
Ingredients:
- 12 prawns, cleaned and deveined
- Salt and ground black pepper, to taste
- ½ tsp. cumin powder
- 1 tsp. fresh lemon juice
- 1 medium egg, whisked
- ⅓ cup of beer
- ½ cup flour
- 1 tsp. baking powder
- 1 tbsp. curry powder
- ½ tsp. grated fresh ginger
- 1 cup flaked coconut

Directions:
1. Coat the prawns in the salt, pepper, cumin powder, and lemon juice.
2. In a bowl, combine together the whisked egg, beer, a quarter-cup of the flour, baking powder, curry, and ginger.
3. In a second bowl, put the remaining quarter-cup of flour, and in a third bowl, the flaked coconut.
4. Dredge the prawns in the flour, before coating them in the beer mixture. Finally, coat your prawns in the flaked coconut.
5. Air-fry at 360°F for 5 minutes. Flip them and allow to cook on the other side for another 2 to 3 minutes before serving.

SNACKS & APPETIZERS RECIPES

218.Old-fashioned Onion Rings

Servings:4
Cooking Time:10 Minutes
Ingredients:

- 1 large onion, cut into rings
- 1¼ cups all-purpose flour
- 1 cup milk
- 1 egg
- ¾ cup dry bread crumbs
- Salt, to taste

Directions:

1. Preheat the Air fryer to 360 °F and grease the Air fryer basket.
2. Mix together flour and salt in a dish.
3. Whisk egg with milk in a second dish until well mixed.
4. Place the breadcrumbs in a third dish.
5. Coat the onion rings with the flour mixture and dip into the egg mixture.
6. Lastly dredge in the breadcrumbs and transfer the onion rings in the Air fryer basket.
7. Cook for about 10 minutes and dish out to serve warm.

219.Cheese Boats

Servings: 2
Cooking Time: 30 Minutes
Ingredients:

- 1 cup ground chicken
- 1 zucchini
- 1 ½ cups crushed tomatoes
- ½ tsp. salt
- ¼ tsp. pepper
- ½ tsp. garlic powder
- 2 tbsp. butter or olive oil
- ½ cup cheese, grated
- ¼ tsp. dried oregano

Directions:

1. 1 Peel and halve the zucchini. Use a spoon to scoop out the flesh.
2. 2 In a bowl, combine the ground chicken, tomato, garlic powder, butter, cheese, oregano, salt, and pepper. Fill in the hollowed-out zucchini with this mixture.
3. 3 Transfer to the Air Fryer and bake for about 10 minutes at 400°F. Serve warm.

220.Asparagus Fries

Servings: 5
Cooking Time: 10 Minutes
Ingredients:

- 1 lb asparagus spears
- 1 cup pork rinds, crushed
- 1/4 cup almond flour
- 2 eggs, lightly beaten
- 1/2 cup parmesan cheese, grated
- Pepper
- Salt

Directions:

1. Preheat the air fryer to 380 F.
2. In a small bowl, mix together parmesan cheese, almond flour, pepper, and salt.
3. In a shallow bowl, whisk eggs.
4. Add crushed pork rind into the shallow dish.
5. Spray air fryer basket with cooking spray.
6. First coat asparagus with parmesan mixture then into the eggs and finally coat with crushed pork rind.
7. Place coated asparagus into the air fryer basket and cook for 10 minutes.
8. Serve and enjoy.

221.Broccoli Pop-corn

Servings: 4
Cooking Time: 6 Minutes
Ingredients:

- 2 cups broccoli florets
- 2 cups coconut flour
- 1/4 cup butter, melted
- 4 eggs yolks
- Pepper
- Salt

Directions:

1. In a bowl whisk egg yolk with melted butter, pepper, and salt. Add coconut flour and stir to combine.
2. Preheat the air fryer to 400 F.
3. Spray air fryer basket with cooking spray.
4. Coat each broccoli floret with egg mixture and place into the air fryer basket and cook for 6 minutes.
5. Serve and enjoy.

222.Spicy Avocado Fries Wrapped In Bacon

Servings: 5
Cooking Time: 10 Minutes
Ingredients:

- 2 teaspoons chili powder
- 2 avocados, pitted and cut into 10 pieces
- 1 teaspoon salt
- ½ teaspoon garlic powder
- 1 teaspoon ground black pepper
- 5 rashers back bacon, cut into halves

Directions:

1. Lay the bacon rashers on a clean surface; then, place one piece of avocado slice on each bacon slice. Add the salt, black pepper, chili powder, and garlic powder.

2. Then, wrap the bacon slice around the avocado and repeat with the remaining rolls; secure them with a cocktail sticks or toothpicks.
3. Preheat your Air Fryer to 370 degrees F; cook in the preheated air fryer for 5 minutes and serve with your favorite sauce for dipping.

223.Cheese Pastries

Servings:6
Cooking Time: 5 Minutes
Ingredients:

- 1 egg yolk
- 4 ounces feta cheese, crumbled
- 1 scallion, finely chopped
- 2 tablespoons fresh parsley, finely chopped
- Salt and ground black pepper, as needed
- 2 frozen filo pastry sheets, thawed
- 2 tablespoons olive oil

Directions:

1. In a large bowl, add the egg yolk, and beat well.
2. Add in the feta cheese, scallion, parsley, salt, and black pepper. Mix well.
3. Cut each filo pastry sheet in three strips.
4. Add about 1 teaspoon of feta mixture on the underside of a strip.
5. Fold the tip of sheet over the filling in a zigzag manner to form a triangle.
6. Repeat with the remaining strips and fillings.
7. Set the temperature of Air Fryer to 390 degrees F.
8. Coat each pastry evenly with oil.
9. Place the pastries in an Air Fryer basket in a single layer.

10. Air Fry for about 3 minutes, then air fryer for about 2 minutes on 360 degrees F.
11. Serve.

224.Herb-roasted Cauliflower

Servings: 2
Cooking Time: 20 Minutes
Ingredients:
- 3 cups cauliflower florets
- 2 tablespoons sesame oil
- 1 teaspoon onion powder
- 1 teaspoon garlic powder
- 1 teaspoon thyme
- 1 teaspoon sage
- 1 teaspoon rosemary
- Sea salt and cracked black pepper, to taste
- 1 teaspoon paprika

Directions:
1. Start by preheating your Air Fryer to 400 degrees F.
2. Toss the cauliflower with the remaining ingredients; toss to coat well.
3. Cook for 12 minutes, shaking the cooking basket halfway through the cooking time. They will crisp up as they cool. Bon appétit!

225.Ham & Cheese Rolls

Servings: 4
Cooking Time: 5 Minutes
Ingredients:
- 16 slices ham
- 1 package chive and onion cream cheese (8 oz)
- 16 slices thin Swiss cheese

Directions:
1. Place the ham on a chopping board.
2. Dry the slices with a paper towel.
3. Thinly spread 2 teaspoons of Swiss cheese over each slice of ham.
4. On the clean section of ham, add a half inch slice of cheese.
5. On the cheese side, fold the ham over the cheese and roll it up.
6. Leave it as is, or slice into smaller rolls.

226.Cucumber And Spring Onions Salsa

Servings: 4
Cooking Time: 5 Minutes
Ingredients:
- 1 and ½ pounds cucumbers, sliced
- 2 spring onions, chopped
- 2 tomatoes cubed
- 2 red chili peppers, chopped
- 2 tablespoons ginger, grated
- 1 tablespoon balsamic vinegar
- A drizzle of olive oil

Directions:
1. In a pan that fits your air fryer, mix all the ingredients, toss, introduce in the fryer and cook at 340 degrees F for 5 minutes. Divide into bowls and serve cold as an appetizer.

227.Chives Salmon Dip

Servings: 4
Cooking Time: 6 Minutes
Ingredients:
- 8 ounces cream cheese, soft
- 2 tablespoons lemon juice
- ½ cup coconut cream
- 4 ounces smoked salmon, skinless, boneless and minced
- A pinch of salt and black pepper
- 1 tablespoon chives, chopped

Directions:
1. In a bowl, mix all the ingredients and whisk them really well. Transfer the mix to a ramekin, place it in your air

fryer's basket and cook at 360 degrees F for 6 minutes. Serve as a party spread.

228.Lemon Green Beans

Servings: 4
Cooking Time: 20 Minutes
Ingredients:

- 1 lemon, juiced
- 1 lb. green beans, washed and destemmed
- ¼ tsp. extra virgin olive oil
- Sea salt to taste
- Black pepper to taste

Directions:

1. Pre-heat the Air Fryer to 400°F.
2. Put the green beans in your Air Fryer basket and drizzle the lemon juice over them.
3. Sprinkle on the pepper and salt. Pour in the oil, and toss to coat the green beans well.
4. Cook for 10 – 12 minutes and serve warm.

229.Puerto Rican Tostones

Servings: 2
Cooking Time: 15 Minutes
Ingredients:

- 1 ripe plantain, sliced
- 1 tablespoon sunflower oil
- A pinch of grated nutmeg
- A pinch of kosher salt

Directions:

1. Toss the plantains with the oil, nutmeg, and salt in a bowl.
2. Cook in the preheated Air Fryer at 400 degrees F for 10 minutes, shaking the cooking basket halfway through the cooking time.
3. Adjust the seasonings to taste and serve immediately.

230.Stuffed Eggs

Servings:4
Cooking Time: 17 Minutes
Ingredients:

- 4 eggs
- 2 oz avocado, peeled, mashed
- 1 teaspoon lemon juice
- ¼ teaspoon butter, melted

Directions:

1. Place the eggs in the air fryer and cook them at 250F for 17 minutes. Then cool and peel the eggs. Cut the eggs into halves and remove the egg yolk. Churn the egg yolks with the help of the fork. Add butter, mashed avocado, and lemon juice. Stir the mixture until smooth. Fill the egg whites with the avocado mixture.

231.Cheese Filled Bell Peppers

Servings:3
Cooking Time:12 Minutes
Ingredients:

- 1 small green bell pepper
- 1 small red bell pepper
- 1 small yellow bell pepper
- ½ cup mozzarella cheese
- ½ cup cream cheese
- 3 teaspoons red chili flakes

Directions:

1. Preheat the Air fryer to 320 °F and grease an Air fryer basket.
2. Chop the tops of the bell peppers and remove all the seeds.
3. Mix together mozzarella cheese, cream cheese and red chili flakes in a bowl.
4. Stuff this cheese mixture in the bell peppers and put back the tops.
5. Arrange in the Air Fryer basket and cook for about 12 minutes.

6. Remove from the Air fryer and serve hot.

232.Healthy Tofu Steaks

Servings: 4
Cooking Time: 35 Minutes
Ingredients:
- 1 package tofu, press and remove excess liquid
- 1/4 tsp dried thyme
- 1/4 cup lemon juice
- 2 tbsp lemon zest
- 3 garlic cloves, minced
- 1/4 cup olive oil
- Pepper
- Salt

Directions:
1. Cut tofu into eight pieces.
2. In a bowl, mix together olive oil, thyme, lemon juice, lemon zest, garlic, pepper, and salt.
3. Add tofu into the bowl and coat well and place in the refrigerator for overnight.
4. Spray air fryer basket with cooking spray.
5. Place marinated tofu into the air fryer basket and cook at 350 F for 30-35 minutes. Turn halfway through.
6. Serve and enjoy.

233.Broccoli Bites

Servings:10
Cooking Time:12 Minutes
Ingredients:
- 2 cups broccoli florets
- 2 eggs, beaten
- 1¼ cups cheddar cheese, grated
- ¼ cup Parmesan cheese, grated
- 1¼ cups panko breadcrumbs
- Salt and black pepper, to taste

Directions:

1. Preheat the Air fryer to 350 °F and grease an Air fryer basket.
2. Mix broccoli with rest of the ingredients and mix until well combined.
3. Make small equal-sized balls from mixture and arrange these balls on a baking sheet.
4. Refrigerate for about half an hour and then transfer into the Air fryer basket.
5. Cook for about 12 minutes and dish out to serve warm.

234.Crispy Cauliflower Poppers

Servings:4
Cooking Time:20 Minutes
Ingredients:
- 1 large egg white
- ¾ cup panko breadcrumbs
- 4 cups cauliflower florets
- 3 tablespoons ketchup
- 2 tablespoons hot sauce

Directions:
1. Preheat the Air fryer to 320 °F and grease an Air fryer basket.
2. Mix together the egg white, ketchup, and hot sauce in a bowl until well combined.
3. Stir in the cauliflower florets and generously coat with marinade.
4. Place breadcrumbs in a shallow dish and dredge the cauliflower florets in it.
5. Arrange the cauliflower florets in the Air fryer basket and cook for about 20 minutes, flipping once in between.
6. Dish out and serve warm.

235.Avocado Wedges

Servings: 4
Cooking Time: 8 Minutes
Ingredients:

- 4 avocados, peeled, pitted and cut into wedges
- 1 egg, whisked
- 1 and ½ cups almond meal
- A pinch of salt and black pepper
- Cooking spray

Directions:
1. Put the egg in a bowl, and the almond meal in another. Season avocado wedges with salt and pepper, coat them in egg and then in meal almond. Arrange the avocado bites in your air fryer's basket, grease them with cooking spray and cook at 400 degrees F for 8 minutes. Serve as a snack right away.

236.Chicken And Berries Bowls

Servings: 2
Cooking Time: 20 Minutes
Ingredients:
- 1 chicken breast, skinless, boneless and cut into strips
- 2 cups baby spinach
- 1 cup blueberries
- 6 strawberries, chopped
- ½ cup walnuts, chopped
- 3 tablespoons balsamic vinegar
- 1 tablespoon olive oil
- 3 tablespoons feta cheese, crumbled

Directions:
1. Heat up a pan that fits the air fryer with the oil over medium heat, add the meat and brown it for 5 minutes. Add the rest of the ingredients except the spinach, toss, introduce in the fryer and cook at 370 degrees F for 15 minutes. Add the spinach, toss, cook for another 5 minutes, divide into bowls and serve.

237.Cajun Cheese Sticks

Servings: 4
Cooking Time: 15 Minutes
Ingredients:
- 1/2 cup all-purpose flour
- 2 eggs
- 1/2 cup parmesan cheese, grated
- 1 tablespoon Cajun seasonings
- 8 cheese sticks, kid-friendly
- 1/4 cup ketchup

Directions:
1. To begin, set up your breading station. Place the all-purpose flour in a shallow dish. In a separate dish, whisk the eggs.
2. Finally, mix the parmesan cheese and Cajun seasoning in a third dish.
3. Start by dredging the cheese sticks in the flour; then, dip them into the egg. Press the cheese sticks into the parmesan mixture, coating evenly.
4. Place the breaded cheese sticks in the lightly greased Air Fryer basket. Cook at 380 degrees F for 6 minutes.
5. Serve with ketchup and enjoy!

238.Cilantro Pork Meatballs

Servings: 12
Cooking Time: 20 Minutes
Ingredients:
- 1 pound pork meat, ground
- 3 spring onions, minced
- 3 tablespoons cilantro, chopped
- 1 tablespoon ginger, grated
- 2 garlic cloves, minced
- 1 chili pepper, minced
- A pinch of salt and black pepper
- 1 and ½ tablespoons coconut aminos
- Cooking spray

Directions:

1. In a bowl, mix all the ingredients except the cooking spray, stir really well and shape medium meatballs out of this mix. Arrange them in your air fryer's basket, grease with cooking spray and cook at 380 degrees F for 20 minutes. Serve as an appetizer.

239.Cabbage Chips

Servings: 6
Cooking Time: 30 Minutes
Ingredients:
- 1 large cabbage head, tear cabbage leaves into pieces
- 2 tbsp olive oil
- 1/4 cup parmesan cheese, grated
- Pepper
- Salt

Directions:
1. Preheat the air fryer to 250 F.
2. Add all ingredients into the large mixing bowl and toss well.
3. Spray air fryer basket with cooking spray.
4. Divide cabbage in batches.
5. Add one cabbage chips batch in air fryer basket and cook for 25-30 minutes at 250 F or until chips are crispy and lightly golden brown.
6. Serve and enjoy.

240.Spinach Dip

Servings:8
Cooking Time: 40 Minutes
Ingredients:
- 8 oz cream cheese, softened
- 1/4 tsp garlic powder
- 1/2 cup onion, minced
- 1/3 cup water chestnuts, drained and chopped
- 1 cup mayonnaise
- 1 cup parmesan cheese, grated
- 1 cup frozen spinach, thawed and squeeze out all liquid
- 1/2 tsp pepper

Directions:
1. Spray air fryer baking dish with cooking spray.
2. Add all ingredients into the bowl and mix until well combined.
3. Transfer bowl mixture into the prepared baking dish and place dish in air fryer basket.
4. Cook at 300 F for 35-40 minutes. After 20 minutes of cooking stir dip.
5. Serve and enjoy.

241.Rice Bites

Servings:4
Cooking Time: 20 Minutes
Ingredients:
- 3 cups cooked risotto
- 1/3 cup Parmesan cheese, grated
- 1 egg, beaten
- 3 ounces mozzarella cheese, cubed
- ¾ cup breadcrumbs

Directions:
1. In a bowl, mix together the risotto, Parmesan cheese, and egg.
2. Make 20 equal-sized balls from the mixture.
3. Insert a mozzarella cube in the center of each ball and using your fingers, smooth the risotto mixture to cover the mozzarella.
4. In a shallow dish, add the breadcrumbs.
5. Coat the balls evenly with breadcrumbs.
6. Set the temperature of Air Fryer to 390 degrees F.
7. Arrange the balls in an Air Fryer basket in a single layer in 2 batches.

8. Air Fry for about 10 minutes or until they turn golden brown.
9. Serve.

242.Bacon Fries

Servings: 2 – 4
Cooking Time: 60 Minutes
Ingredients:
- 2 large russet potatoes, peeled and cut into ½ inch sticks
- 5 slices of bacon, diced
- 2 tbsp. vegetable oil
- 2 ½ cups cheddar cheese, shredded
- 3 oz. cream cheese, melted
- Salt and freshly ground black pepper
- ¼ cup chopped scallions
- Ranch dressing

Directions:
1. 1 Boil a large pot of salted water.
2. 2 Briefly cook the potato sticks in the boiling water for 4 minutes.
3. 3 Drain the potatoes and run some cold water over them in order to wash off the starch. Pat them dry with a kitchen towel.
4. 4 Pre-heat the Air Fryer to 400°F.
5. 5 Put the chopped bacon in the Air Fryer and air-fry for 4 minutes. Shake the basket at the halfway point.
6. 6 Place the bacon on paper towels to drain any excess fat and remove the grease from the Air Fryer drawer.
7. 7 Coat the dried potatoes with oil and put them in the Air Fryer basket. Air-fry at 360°F for 25 minutes, giving the basket the occasional shake throughout the cooking time and sprinkling the fries with salt and freshly ground black pepper at the halfway point.
8. 8 Take a casserole dish or baking pan that is small enough to fit inside your Air Fryer and place the fries inside.
9. 9 Mix together the 2 cups of the Cheddar cheese and the melted cream cheese.
10. 10 Pour the cheese mixture over the fries and top them with the rest of the Cheddar cheese and the cooked bacon crumbles.
11. 11 Take absolute care when placing the baking pan inside the cooker. Use a foil sling [a sheet of aluminum foil folded into a strip about 2 inches wide by 24 inches long].
12. 12 Cook the fries at 340°F for 5 minutes, ensuring the cheese melts.
13. 13 Garnish the fries with the chopped scallions and serve straight from in the baking dish with some ranch dressing.

243.Tomato Salad

Servings: 6
Cooking Time: 12 Minutes
Ingredients:
- 1 pound tomatoes, sliced
- 1 tablespoon balsamic vinegar
- 1 tablespoon ginger, grated
- ½ teaspoon coriander, ground
- 1 teaspoon sweet paprika
- 1 teaspoon chili powder
- 1 cup mozzarella, shredded

Directions:
1. In a pan that fits your air fryer, mix all the ingredients except the mozzarella, toss, introduce the pan in the air fryer and cook at 360 degrees F for 12 minutes. Divide into bowls and serve cold as an appetizer with the mozzarella sprinkled all over.

244.Fruit Pastries

Servings:8

Cooking Time: 20 Minutes

Ingredients:

- ½ of apple, peeled, cored and chopped
- 1 teaspoon fresh orange zest, finely grated
- ½ tablespoon white sugar
- ½ teaspoon ground cinnamon
- 7.05 ounces prepared frozen puff pastry

Directions:

1. In a bowl, mix together all the ingredients except puff pastry.
2. Cut the pastry in 16 squares.
3. Using a teaspoon, place apple mixture in the center of each square.
4. Fold each square into a triangle and slightly press the edges with your wet fingers.
5. Then, using a fork, firmly press the edges.
6. Set the temperature of Air Fryer to 390 degrees F.
7. Add the pastries into an Air Fryer basket in a single layer in 2 batches.
8. Air Fry for about 10 minutes.
9. Enjoy!

245.Creamy Cheddar Eggs

Servings:8

Cooking Time: 16 Minutes

Ingredients:

- 4 eggs
- 2 oz pork rinds
- ¼ cup Cheddar cheese, shredded
- 1 tablespoon heavy cream
- 1 teaspoon fresh dill, chopped

Directions:

1. Place the eggs in the air fryer and cook them at 255F for 16 minutes. Then cool the eggs in the cold water and peel. Cut every egg into the halves and remove the egg yolks. Transfer the egg yolks in the mixing bowl. Add shredded cheese, heavy cream, and fresh dill. Stir the mixture with the help of the fork until smooth and add pork rinds. Mix it up. Fill the egg whites with the egg yolk mixture.

246.Broccoli Melts With Coriander And Cheese

Servings: 6

Cooking Time: 20 Minutes

Ingredients:

- 2 eggs, well whisked
- 2 cups Colby cheese, shredded
- 1/2 cup almond meal
- 2 tablespoons sesame seeds
- Seasoned salt, to taste
- 1/4 teaspoon ground black pepper, or more to taste
- 1 head broccoli, grated
- 1 cup parmesan cheese, grated

Directions:

1. Thoroughly combine the eggs, Colby cheese, almond meal, sesame seeds, salt, black pepper, and broccoli to make the consistency of dough.
2. Chill for 1 hour and shape into small balls; roll the patties over parmesan cheese. Spritz them with cooking oil on all sides.
3. Cook at 360 degrees F for 10 minutes. Check for doneness and return to the Air Fryer for 8 to 10 more minutes. Serve with a sauce for dipping. Bon appétit!

247.Buffalo Cauliflower

Servings: 1
Cooking Time: 10 Minutes
Ingredients:
- ½ packet dry ranch seasoning
- 2 tbsp. salted butter, melted
- Cauliflower florets
- ¼ cup buffalo sauce

Directions:
1. In a bowl, combine the dry ranch seasoning and butter. Toss with the cauliflower florets to coat and transfer them to the fryer.
2. Cook at 400°F for five minutes, shaking the basket occasionally to ensure the florets cook evenly.
3. Remove the cauliflower from the fryer, pour the buffalo sauce over it, and enjoy.

248.Broccoli And Pecorino Toscano Fat Bombs

Servings: 6
Cooking Time: 20 Minutes
Ingredients:
- 1 large-sized head of broccoli, broken into small florets
- 1/2 teaspoon sea salt
- 1/4 teaspoon ground black pepper, or more to taste
- 1 tablespoon Shoyu sauce
- 1 teaspoon groundnut oil
- 1 cup bacon bits
- 1 cup Pecorino Toscano, freshly grated
- Paprika, to taste

Directions:
1. Add the broccoli florets to boiling water; boil approximately 4 minutes; drain well.
2. Season with salt and pepper; drizzle with Shoyu sauce and groundnut oil. Mash with a potato masher.
3. Add the bacon and cheese to the mixture; shape the mixture into bite-sized balls.
4. Air-fry at 390 degrees F for 10 minutes; shake the Air Fryer basket, push the power button again, and continue to cook for 5 minutes more.
5. Toss the fried keto bombs with paprika. Bon appétit!

DESSERTS RECIPES

249.Raspberry-coco Desert

Servings:12
Cooking Time: 20 Minutes
Ingredients:
- ¼ cup coconut oil
- 1 cup coconut milk
- 1 cup raspberries, pulsed
- 1 teaspoon vanilla bean
- 1/3 cup erythritol powder
- 3 cups desiccated coconut

Directions:
1. Preheat the air fryer for 5 minutes.
2. Combine all ingredients in a mixing bowl.
3. Pour into a greased baking dish.
4. Bake in the air fryer for 20 minutes at 375 °F.

250.Cranberry Cream Surprise

Servings: 1
Cooking Time: 30 Minutes
Ingredients:
- 1 cup mashed cranberries
- ½ cup Confectioner's Style Swerve
- 2 tsp natural cherry flavoring
- 2 tsp natural rum flavoring
- 1 cup organic heavy cream

Directions:
1. Combine the mashed cranberries, sweetener, cherry and rum flavorings.
2. Cover and refrigerate for 20 minutes.
3. Whip the heavy cream until soft peaks form.
4. Layer the whipped cream and cranberry mixture.
5. Top with fresh cranberries, mint leaves or grated dark chocolate.
6. Serve!

251.Chocolate Cake

Servings:4
Cooking Time: 40 Minutes
Ingredients:
- For Cake:
- 1/3 cup plain flour
- ¼ teaspoon baking powder
- 1½ tablespoons unsweetened cocoa powder
- 2 egg yolks
- ½ ounce caster sugar
- 2 tablespoons vegetable oil
- 3¾ tablespoons milk
- 1 teaspoon vanilla extract
- For Meringue:
- 2 egg whites
- 1 ounce caster sugar
- 1/8 teaspoon cream of tartar

Directions:
1. For cake: in a bowl, sift together the flour, baking powder, and cocoa powder.
2. In another bowl, add the remaining ingredients and whisk until well combined.
3. Add the flour mixture and whisk until well combined.
4. For meringue: in a clean glass bowl, add all the ingredients and with an electric whisker, whisk on high speed until stiff peaks form.
5. Place 1/3 of the meringue into flour mixture and with a hand whisker, whisk well.
6. Fold in the remaining meringue.
7. Set the temperature of air fryer to 355 degrees F.
8. Place the mixture into an ungreased chiffon pan.

9. With a piece of foil, cover the pan tightly and poke some holes using a fork.
10. Arrange the cake pan into an air fryer basket.
11. Now, set the temperature of air fryer to 320 degrees F.
12. Air fry for about 30-35 minutes.
13. Remove the piece of foil and set the temperature to 285 degrees F.
14. Air fry for another 5 minutes or until a toothpick inserted in the center comes out clean.
15. Remove the cake pan from air fryer and place onto a wire rack to cool for about 10 minutes.
16. Now, invert the cake onto wire rack to completely cool before slicing.
17. Cut the cake into desired size slices and serve.

252.Lemon Butter Bars

Servings: 8
Cooking Time: 35 Minutes
Ingredients:
- ½ cup butter, melted
- 1 cup erythritol
- 1 and ¾ cups almond flour
- 3 eggs, whisked
- Zest of 1 lemon, grated
- Juice of 3 lemons

Directions:
1. In a bowl, mix 1 cup flour with half of the erythritol and the butter, stir well and press into a baking dish that fits the air fryer lined with parchment paper. Put the dish in your air fryer and cook at 350 degrees F for 10 minutes. Meanwhile, in a bowl, mix the rest of the flour with the remaining erythritol and the other

ingredients and whisk well. Spread this over the crust, put the dish in the air fryer once more and cook at 350 degrees F for 25 minutes. Cool down, cut into bars and serve.

253.Easy Chocolate And Coconut Cake

Servings: 10
Cooking Time: 20 Minutes
Ingredients:
- 1 stick butter
- 1 ¼ cups dark chocolate, broken into chunks
- 1/4 cup tablespoon agave syrup
- 1/4 cup sugar
- 2 tablespoons milk
- 2 eggs, beaten
- 1/3 cup coconut, shredded

Directions:
1. Begin by preheating your Air Fryer to 330 degrees F.
2. In a microwave-safe bowl, melt the butter, chocolate, and agave syrup. Allow it to cool to room temperature.
3. Add the remaining ingredients to the chocolate mixture; stir to combine well. Scrape the batter into a lightly greased baking pan.
4. Bake in the preheated Air Fryer for 15 minutes or until a toothpick comes out dry and clean. Enjoy!

254.Cardamom Bombs

Servings: 2
Cooking Time: 5 Minutes
Ingredients:
- 2 oz avocado, peeled
- 1 egg, beaten
- ½ teaspoon ground cardamom
- 1 tablespoon Erythritol
- 2 tablespoons coconut flour
- 1 teaspoon butter, softened

Directions:

1. Put the avocado in the bowl and mash it with the help of the fork. Add egg and stir the mixture until it is smooth. Then add ground cardamom, Erythritol, and coconut flour. After this, add butter and stir the mixture well. Make the balls from the avocado mixture and press them gently. Then preheat the air fryer to 400F. Put the avocado bombs in the air fryer and cook them for 5 minutes.

255.Classic Mini Cheesecakes

Servings: 8
Cooking Time: 30 Minutes
Ingredients:

- 1/3 teaspoon grated nutmeg
- 1 ½ tablespoons erythritol
- 1 ½ cups almond meal
- 8 tablespoons melted butter
- 1 teaspoon ground cinnamon
- A pinch of kosher salt
- For the Cheesecake:
- 2 eggs
- 1/2 cups unsweetened chocolate chips
- 1 ½ tablespoons sour cream
- 4 ounces soft cheese
- 1/2 cup swerve
- 1/2 teaspoon vanilla essence

Directions:

1. Firstly, line eight cups of mini muffin pan with paper liners.
2. To make the crust, mix the almond meal together with erythritol, cinnamon, nutmeg, and kosher salt.
3. Now, add melted butter and stir well to moisten the crumb mixture.

4. Divide the crust mixture among the muffin cups and press gently to make even layers.
5. In another bowl, whip together the soft cheese, sour cream and swerve until uniform and smooth. Fold in the eggs and the vanilla essence.
6. Then, divide chocolate chips among the prepared muffin cups. Then, add the cheese mix to each muffin cup.
7. Bake for about 18 minutes at 345 degrees F. Bake in batches if needed. To finish, transfer the mini cheesecakes to a cooling rack; store in the fridge.

256.Chocolate Custard

Servings: 4
Cooking Time: 32 Minutes
Ingredients:

- 2 eggs
- 1 tsp vanilla
- 1 cup heavy whipping cream
- 1 cup unsweetened almond milk
- 2 tbsp unsweetened cocoa powder
- 1/4 cup Swerve
- Pinch of salt

Directions:

1. Preheat the air fryer to 305 F.
2. Add all ingredients into the blender and blend until well combined.
3. Pour mixture into the ramekins and place into the air fryer.
4. Cook for 32 minutes.
5. Serve and enjoy.

257.Bananas & Ice Cream

Servings: 2
Cooking Time: 25 Minutes
Ingredients:

- 2 large bananas
- 1 tbsp. butter

- 1 tbsp. sugar
- 2 tbsp. friendly bread crumbs
- Vanilla ice cream for serving

Directions:
1. Place the butter in the Air Fryer basket and allow it to melt for 1 minute at 350°F.
2. Combine the sugar and bread crumbs in a bowl.
3. Slice the bananas into 1-inch-round pieces. Drop them into the sugar mixture and coat them well.
4. Place the bananas in the Air Fryer and cook for 10 – 15 minutes.
5. Serve warm, with ice cream on the side if desired.

258.Avocado Chocolate Brownies

Servings: 12
Cooking Time: 30 Minutes
Ingredients:
- 1 cup avocado, peeled and mashed
- ½ teaspoon vanilla extract
- 4 tablespoons cocoa powder
- 3 tablespoons coconut oil, melted
- 2 eggs, whisked
- ½ cup dark chocolate, unsweetened and melted
- ¾ cup almond flour
- 1 teaspoon baking powder
- ¼ teaspoon baking soda
- 1 teaspoon stevia

Directions:
1. In a bowl, mix the flour with stevia, baking powder and soda and stir. Add the rest of the ingredients gradually, whisk and pour into a cake pan that fits the air fryer after you lined it with parchment paper. Put the pan in your air fryer and cook at 350 degrees F

for 30 minutes. Cut into squares and serve cold.

259.Glazed Donuts

Servings: 2 – 4
Cooking Time: 25 Minutes
Ingredients:
- 1 can [8 oz.] refrigerated croissant dough
- Cooking spray
- 1 can [16 oz.] vanilla frosting

Directions:
1. Cut the croissant dough into 1-inch-round slices. Make a hole in the center of each one to create a donut.
2. Put the donuts in the Air Fryer basket, taking care not to overlap any, and spritz with cooking spray. You may need to cook everything in multiple batches.
3. Cook at 400°F for 2 minutes. Turn the donuts over and cook for another 3 minutes.
4. Place the rolls on a paper plate.
5. Microwave a half-cup of frosting for 30 seconds and pour a drizzling of the frosting over the donuts before serving.

260.Butter Rum Cookies With Walnuts

Servings: 6
Cooking Time: 35 Minutes
Ingredients:
- 1 cup all-purpose flour
- 1/2 teaspoon baking powder
- 1/4 teaspoon fine sea salt
- 1 stick butter, unsalted and softened
- 1/2 cup sugar
- 1 egg
- 1/2 teaspoon vanilla
- 1 teaspoon butter rum flavoring
- 3 ounces walnuts, finely chopped

Directions:

1. Begin by preheating the Air Fryer to 360 degrees F.
2. In a mixing dish, thoroughly combine the flour with baking powder and salt.
3. Beat the butter and sugar with a hand mixer until pale and fluffy; add the whisked egg, vanilla, and butter rum flavoring; mix again to combine well. Now, stir in the dry ingredients.
4. Fold in the chopped walnuts and mix to combine. Divide the mixture into small balls; flatten each ball with a fork and transfer them to a foil-lined baking pan.
5. Bake in the preheated Air Fryer for 14 minutes. Work in a few batches and transfer to wire racks to cool completely. Bon appétit!

261.Rich Layered Cake

Servings:8
Cooking Time:25 Minutes
Ingredients:

- For Cake:
- 3½-ounce plain flour
- 3½-ounce butter, softened
- 2 medium eggs
- For Filling:
- 1¾-ounce butter, softened
- 2 tablespoons strawberry jam
- For Cake:
- 1 teaspoon ground cinnamon
- Pinch of salt
- 7 tablespoons sugar
- For Filling:
- 1 tablespoon whipped cream
- 2/3 cup icing sugar

Directions:

1. Preheat the Air fryer to 355 °F and grease a cake pan lightly.

2. For Cake:
3. Mix flour, cinnamon and salt in a large bowl.
4. Beat together sugar, eggs and butter in another bowl until creamy.
5. Stir in the flour mixture slowly and beat until well combined
6. Transfer the mixture into the cake pan and cook for about 15 minutes.
7. Set the Air fryer to 335 degrees F and cook for about 10 minutes.
8. Remove the cake from the Air fryer and cut the cake in 2 portions.
9. For Filling:
10. Mix butter, cream and icing sugar in a bowl and beat until creamy.
11. Place 1 cake portion in a plate, cut side up and spread jam evenly over cake.
12. Top with the butter mixture and place another cake, cut side down over filling to serve.

262.Delicious Fall Clafoutis

Servings:6
Cooking Time:30 Minutes
Ingredients:

- 3/4 cup extra-fine flour
- 1 ½ cups plums, pitted and
- 4 medium-sized pears, cored and sliced
- 1/2 cup coconut cream
- 3/4 cup coconut milk
- 3 eggs, whisked
- 1/2 cup powdered sugar, for dusting
- 3/4 cup white sugar
- 1/2 teaspoon baking soda
- 1/2 teaspoon baking powder
- 1/3 teaspoon ground cinnamon
- 1/2 teaspoon crystalized ginger
- 1/4 teaspoon grated nutmeg

Directions:

1. Lightly grease 2 mini pie pans using a nonstick cooking spray. Lay the plums and pears on the bottom of the pie pans.
2. In a saucepan that is preheated over a moderate flame, warm the cream along with coconut milk until thoroughly heated.
3. Remove the pan from the heat; mix in the flour along with baking soda and baking powder.
4. In a medium-sized mixing bowl, whip the eggs, white sugar, and spices; whip until the mixture is creamy.
5. Add the creamy milk mixture. Carefully spread this mixture over the fruits.
6. Bake at 320 degrees for about 25 minutes. To serve, dust with powdered sugar.

263.Chocolate Cheesecake

Servings: 4
Cooking Time: 60 Minutes
Ingredients:

- 4 oz cream cheese
- ½ oz heavy cream
- 1 tsp Sugar Glycerite
- 1 tsp Splenda
- 1 oz Enjoy Life mini chocolate chips

Directions:

1. Combine all the ingredients except the chocolate to a thick consistency.
2. Fold in the chocolate chips.
3. Refrigerate in serving cups.
4. Serve!

264.Butter Crumble

Servings: 4
Cooking Time: 25 Minutes
Ingredients:

- ½ cup coconut flour
- 2 tablespoons butter, softened
- 2 tablespoon Erythritol
- 3 oz peanuts, crushed
- 1 tablespoon cream cheese
- 1 teaspoon baking powder
- ½ teaspoon lemon juice

Directions:

1. In the mixing bowl mix up coconut flour, butter, Erythritol, baking powder, and lemon juice. Stir the mixture until homogenous. Then place it in the freezer for 10 minutes. Meanwhile, mix up peanuts and cream cheese. Grate the frozen dough. Line the air fryer mold with baking paper. Then put ½ of grated dough in the mold and flatten it. Top it with cream cheese mixture. Then put remaining grated dough over the cream cheese mixture. Place the mold with the crumble in the air fryer and cook it for 25 minutes at 330F.

265.Pear Fritters With Cinnamon And Ginger

Servings: 4
Cooking Time: 20 Minutes
Ingredients:

- 2 pears, peeled, cored and sliced
- 1 tablespoon coconut oil, melted
- 1 ½ cups all-purpose flour
- 1 teaspoon baking powder
- A pinch of fine sea salt
- A pinch of freshly grated nutmeg
- 1/2 teaspoon ginger
- 1 teaspoon cinnamon
- 2 eggs
- 4 tablespoons milk

Directions:

1. Mix all ingredients, except for the pears, in a shallow bowl. Dip each slice of the pears in the batter until well coated.
2. Cook in the preheated Air Fryer at 360 degrees for 4 minutes, flipping them halfway through the cooking time. Repeat with the remaining ingredients.
3. Dust with powdered sugar if desired. Bon appétit!

266.Hazelnut Brownie Cups

Servings: 12
Cooking Time: 30 Minutes
Ingredients:
- 6 oz. semisweet chocolate chips
- 1 stick butter, at room temperature
- 1 cup sugar
- 2 large eggs
- ¼ cup red wine
- ¼ tsp. hazelnut extract
- 1 tsp. pure vanilla extract
- ¾ cup flour
- 2 tbsp. cocoa powder
- ½ cup ground hazelnuts
- Pinch of kosher salt

Directions:
1. Melt the butter and chocolate chips in the microwave.
2. In a large bowl, combine the sugar, eggs, red wine, hazelnut and vanilla extract with a whisk. Pour in the chocolate mix.
3. Add in the flour, cocoa powder, ground hazelnuts, and a pinch of kosher salt, continuing to stir until a creamy, smooth consistency is achieved.

4. Take a muffin tin and place a cupcake liner in each cup. Spoon an equal amount of the batter into each one.
5. Air bake at 360°F for 28 - 30 minutes, cooking in batches if necessary.
6. Serve with a topping of ganache if desired.

267.Perfect Apple Pie

Servings:6
Cooking Time:30 Minutes
Ingredients:
- 1 frozen pie crust, thawed
- 1 large apple, peeled, cored and chopped
- 1 tablespoon butter, chopped
- 1 egg, beaten
- 3 tablespoons sugar, divided
- 1 tablespoon ground cinnamon
- 2 teaspoons fresh lemon juice
- ½ teaspoon vanilla extract

Directions:
1. Preheat the Air fryer to 320 °F and grease a pie pan lightly.
2. Cut 2 crusts, first about 1/8-inch larger than pie pan and second, a little smaller than first one.
3. Arrange the large crust in the bottom of pie pan.
4. Mix apple, 2 tablespoons of sugar, cinnamon, lemon juice and vanilla extract in a large bowl.
5. Put the apple mixture evenly over the bottom crust and top with butter.
6. Arrange the second crust on top and seal the edges.
7. Cut 4 slits in the top crust carefully and brush with egg.
8. Sprinkle with sugar and arrange the pie pan in the Air fryer basket.

9. Cook for about 30 minutes and dish out to serve.

268.Rhubarb Pie Recipe

Servings: 6
Cooking Time:1 Hour 15 Minutes
Ingredients:
- 1 ¼ cups almond flour
- 5 tbsp. cold water
- 8 tbsp. butter
- 1 tsp. sugar
- For the filling:
- 3 cups rhubarb; chopped.
- 1/2 tsp. nutmeg; ground
- 1 tbsp. butter
- 3 tbsp. flour
- 1 ½ cups sugar
- 2 eggs
- 2 tbsp. low fat milk

Directions:
1. In a bowl; mix 1 ¼ cups flour with 1 tsp. sugar, 8 tbsp. butter and cold water; stir and knead until you obtain a dough
2. Transfer dough to a floured working surface, shape a disk, flatten, wrap in plastic, keep in the fridge for about 30 minutes; roll and press on the bottom of a pie pan that fits your air fryer
3. In a bowl; mix rhubarb with 1 ½ cups sugar, nutmeg, 3 tbsp. flour and whisk.
4. In another bowl, whisk eggs with milk, add to rhubarb mix, pour the whole mix into the pie crust, introduce in your air fryer and cook at 390 °F, for 45 minutes. Cut and serve it cold

269.Mini Strawberry Pies

Servings: 8
Cooking Time: 15 Minutes

Ingredients:
- 1 cup sugar
- ¼ tsp. ground cloves
- 1/8 tsp. cinnamon powder
- 1 tsp. vanilla extract
- 1 [12-oz.] can biscuit dough
- 12 oz. strawberry pie filling
- ¼ cup butter, melted

Directions:
1. In a bowl, mix together the sugar, cloves, cinnamon, and vanilla.
2. With a rolling pin, roll each piece of the biscuit dough into a flat, round circle.
3. Spoon an equal amount of the strawberry pie filling onto the center of each biscuit.
4. Roll up the dough. Dip the biscuits into the melted butter and coat them with the sugar mixture.
5. Coat with a light brushing of non-stick cooking spray on all sides.
6. Transfer the cookies to the Air Fryer and bake them at 340°F for roughly 10 minutes, or until a golden-brown color is achieved.
7. Allow to cool for 5 minutes before serving.

270.Almond Pudding

Servings: 6
Cooking Time: 20 Minutes
Ingredients:
- 24 ounces cream cheese, soft
- 2 tablespoons almond meal
- ¼ cup erythritol
- 3 eggs, whisked
- 1 tablespoon vanilla extract
- ½ cup heavy cream
- 12 ounces dark chocolate, melted

Directions:
1. In a bowl mix all the ingredients and whisk well. Divide this into 6 ramekins, put them in your air fryer and cook at 320 degrees F for 20

minutes. Keep in the fridge for 1 hour before serving.

271.Strawberry Shake

Servings: 1
Cooking Time: 5 Minutes
Ingredients:
- 3/4 cup coconut milk (from the carton)
- ¼ cup heavy cream
- 7 ice cubes
- 2 tbsp sugar-free strawberry Torani syrup
- ¼ tsp Xanthan Gum

Directions:
1. Combine all the ingredients into blender.
2. Blend for 1-2 minutes.
3. Serve!

272.Chocolate Mug Cake

Servings:1
Cooking Time:13 Minutes
Ingredients:
- ¼ cup self-rising flour
- 1 tablespoon cocoa powder
- 3 tablespoons whole milk
- 5 tablespoons caster sugar
- 3 tablespoons coconut oil

Directions:
1. Preheat the Air fryer to 390 °F and grease a large mug lightly.
2. Mix all the ingredients in a shallow mug until well combined.
3. Arrange the mug into the Air fryer basket and cook for about 13 minutes.
4. Dish out and serve warm.

273.Air Fryer Chocolate Cake

Servings:6
Cooking Time:25 Minutes
Ingredients:
- 3 eggs
- 1 cup almond flour
- 1 stick butter, room temperature
- 1/3 cup cocoa powder
- 1½ teaspoons baking powder

- ½ cup sour cream
- 2/3 cup swerve
- 2 teaspoons vanilla

Directions:
1. Preheat the Air fryer to 360 °F and grease a cake pan lightly.
2. Mix all the ingredients in a bowl and beat well.
3. Pour the batter in the cake pan and transfer into the Air fryer basket.
4. Cook for about 25 minutes and cut into slices to serve.

274.Semolina Cake

Servings:8
Cooking Time:15 Minutes
Ingredients:
- 2½ cups semolina
- 1 cup milk
- 1 cup Greek yogurt
- 2 teaspoons baking powder
- ½ cup walnuts, chopped
- ½ cup vegetable oil
- 1 cup sugar
- Pinch of salt

Directions:
1. Preheat the Air fryer to 360 °F and grease a baking pan lightly.
2. Mix semolina, oil, milk, yogurt and sugar in a bowl until well combined.
3. Cover the bowl and keep aside for about 15 minutes.
4. Stir in the baking soda, baking powder and salt and fold in the walnuts.
5. Transfer the mixture into the baking pan and place in the Air fryer.
6. Cook for about 15 minutes and dish out to serve.

275.Classic Buttermilk Biscuits

Servings:4
Cooking Time:8 Minutes
Ingredients:
- ½ cup cake flour
- 1¼ cups all-purpose flour

- ¾ teaspoon baking powder
- ¼ cup + 2 tablespoons butter, cut into cubes
- ¾ cup buttermilk
- 1 teaspoon granulated sugar
- Salt, to taste

Directions:
1. Preheat the Air fryer to 400 °F and grease a pie pan lightly.
2. Sift together flours, baking soda, baking powder, sugar and salt in a large bowl.
3. Add cold butter and mix until a coarse crumb is formed.
4. Stir in the buttermilk slowly and mix until a dough is formed.
5. Press the dough into ½ inch thickness onto a floured surface and cut out circles with a 1¾-inch round cookie cutter.
6. Arrange the biscuits in a pie pan in a single layer and brush butter on them.
7. Transfer into the Air fryer and cook for about 8 minutes until golden brown.

276.Cobbler

Servings: 4
Cooking Time: 30 Minutes
Ingredients:
- ¼ cup heavy cream
- 1 egg, beaten
- ½ cup almond flour
- 1 teaspoon vanilla extract
- 2 tablespoons butter, softened
- ¼ cup hazelnuts, chopped

Directions:
1. Mix up heavy cream, egg, almond flour, vanilla extract, and butter. Then whisk the mixture gently. Preheat the air fryer to 325F. Line the air fryer pan with baking paper. Pour ½ part of the batter in the baking pan, flatten it gently and top with hazelnuts. Then pour the remaining batter over the hazelnuts and place the pan in the air

fryer. Cook the cobbler for 30 minutes.

277.Lemon Coffee Muffins

Servings: 6
Cooking Time: 11 Minutes
Ingredients:
- 1 cup almond flour
- 3 tablespoons Erythritol
- 1 scoop protein powder
- 1 teaspoon vanilla extract
- 3 tablespoons coconut oil, melted
- 1 egg, beaten
- ½ teaspoon baking powder
- ½ teaspoon instant coffee
- 1 teaspoon lemon juice
- 2 tablespoons heavy cream
- Cooking spray

Directions:
1. In the mixing bowl mix up almond flour, Erythritol, protein powder, vanilla extract, coconut oil, egg, baking powder, instant coffee, lemon juice, and heavy cream. With the help of the immersion blender, whisk the mixture until you get a smooth batter. After this, preheat the air fryer to 360F. Spray the muffin molds with cooking spray. Then fill ½ part of every muffin mold with muffin batter and transfer them in the air fryer basket. Cook the muffins for 11 minutes.

278.Bread Pudding

Servings:2
Cooking Time:12 Minutes
Ingredients:
- 1 cup milk
- 1 egg
- 2 tablespoons raisins, soaked in hot water for about 15 minutes
- 2 bread slices, cut into small cubes
- 1 tablespoon chocolate chips
- 1 tablespoon brown sugar
- ½ teaspoon ground cinnamon

- ¼ teaspoon vanilla extract
- 1 tablespoon sugar

Directions:
1. Preheat the Air fryer to 375 °F and grease a baking dish lightly.
2. Mix milk, egg, brown sugar, cinnamon and vanilla extract until well combined.
3. Stir in the raisins and mix well.
4. Arrange the bread cubes evenly in the baking dish and top with the milk mixture.
5. Refrigerate for about 20 minutes and sprinkle with chocolate chips and sugar.
6. Transfer the baking pan into the Air fryer and cook for about 12 minutes.
7. Dish out and serve immediately.

279.Chocolate And Peanut Butter Fondants

Servings:4
Cooking Time: 25 Minutes
Ingredients:
- ½ cup peanut butter, crunchy
- 2 tbsp butter, diced
- ¼ cup + ¼ cup sugar
- 4 eggs, room temperature
- ⅛ cup flour, sieved
- 1 tsp salt
- ¼ cup water
- Cooking spray

Directions:
1. Make a salted praline to top the chocolate fondant. Add ¼ cup of sugar, 1 tsp of salt and water into a saucepan. Stir and bring it to a boil over low heat. Simmer until the desired color is achieved and reduced. Pour it into a baking tray and leave to cool and harden.
2. Preheat the air fryer to 300 F.
3. Place a pot of water over medium heat and place a heatproof bowl over it. Add in chocolate, butter, and peanut butter. Stir continuously until fully melted, combined, and smooth. Remove the bowl and allow to cool slightly. Add eggs to the chocolate and whisk. Add flour and remaining sugar; mix well.
4. Grease 4 small loaf pans with cooking spray and divide the chocolate mixture between them. Place 2 pans at a time in the basket and cook for 7 minutes. Remove them and serve the fondants with a piece of salted praline.

OTHER AIR FRYER RECIPES

280.Snapper With Gruyere Cheese

Servings: 4
Cooking Time: 25 Minutes
Ingredients:

- 2 tablespoons olive oil
- 1 shallot, thinly sliced
- 2 garlic cloves, minced
- 1 ½ pounds snapper fillets
- Sea salt and ground black pepper, to taste
- 1 teaspoon cayenne pepper
- 1/2 teaspoon dried basil
- 1/2 cup tomato puree
- 1/2 cup white wine
- 1 cup Gruyere cheese, shredded

Directions:

1. Heat 1 tablespoon of olive oil in a saucepan over medium-high heat. Now, cook the shallot and garlic until tender and aromatic.
2. Preheat your Air Fryer to 370 degrees F.
3. Grease a casserole dish with 1 tablespoon of olive oil. Place the snapper fillet in the casserole dish. Season with salt, black pepper, and cayenne pepper. Add the sautéed shallot mixture.
4. Add the basil, tomato puree and wine to the casserole dish. Cook for 10 minutes in the preheated Air Fryer.
5. Top with the shredded cheese and cook an additional 7 minutes. Serve immediately.

281.Omelet With Mushrooms And Peppers

Servings: 2
Cooking Time: 20 Minutes
Ingredients:

- 1 tablespoon olive oil
- 1/2 cup scallions, chopped
- 1 bell pepper, seeded and thinly sliced
- 6 ounces button mushrooms, thinly sliced
- 4 eggs
- 2 tablespoons milk
- Sea salt and freshly ground black pepper, to taste
- 1 tablespoon fresh chives, for serving

Directions:

1. Heat the olive oil in a skillet over medium-high heat. Now, sauté the scallions and peppers until aromatic.
2. Add the mushrooms and continue to cook an additional 3 minutes or until tender. Reserve.
3. Generously grease a baking pan with nonstick cooking spray.
4. Then, whisk the eggs, milk, salt, and black pepper. Spoon into the prepared baking pan.
5. Cook in the preheated Air Fryer at 360 F for 4 minutes. Flip and cook for a further 3 minutes.
6. Place the reserved mushroom filling on one side of the omelet. Fold your omelet in half and slide onto a serving plate. Serve immediately garnished with fresh chives. Bon appétit!

282.Easiest Pork Chops Ever

Servings: 6
Cooking Time: 22 Minutes
Ingredients:

- 1/3 cup Italian breadcrumbs
- Roughly chopped fresh cilantro, to taste
- 2 teaspoons Cajun seasonings

- Nonstick cooking spray
- 2 eggs, beaten
- 3 tablespoons white flour
- 1 teaspoon seasoned salt
- Garlic & onion spice blend, to taste
- 6 pork chops
- 1/3 teaspoon freshly cracked black pepper

Directions:

1. Coat the pork chops with Cajun seasonings, salt, pepper, and the spice blend on all sides.
2. Then, add the flour to a plate. In a shallow dish, whisk the egg until pale and smooth. Place the Italian breadcrumbs in the third bowl.
3. Dredge each pork piece in the flour; then, coat them with the egg; finally, coat them with the breadcrumbs. Spritz them with cooking spray on both sides.
4. Now, air-fry pork chops for about 18 minutes at 345 degrees F; make sure to taste for doneness after first 12 minutes of cooking. Lastly, garnish with fresh cilantro. Bon appétit!

283.Frittata With Turkey Breasts And Cottage Cheese

Servings: 4
Cooking Time: 50 Minutes
Ingredients:

- 1 tablespoon olive oil
- 1 pound turkey breasts, slices
- 6 large-sized eggs
- 3 tablespoons Greek yogurt
- 3 tablespoons Cottage cheese, crumbled
- 1/4 teaspoon ground black pepper
- 1/4 teaspoon red pepper flakes, crushed

- Himalayan salt, to taste
- 1 red bell pepper, seeded and sliced
- 1 green bell pepper, seeded and sliced

Directions:

1. Grease the cooking basket with olive oil. Add the turkey and cook in the preheated Air Fryer at 350 degrees F for 30 minutes, flipping them over halfway through. Cut into bite-sized strips and reserve.
2. Now, beat the eggs with Greek yogurt, cheese, black pepper, red pepper, and salt. Add the bell peppers to a baking pan that is previously lightly greased with a cooking spray.
3. Add the turkey strips; pour the egg mixture over all ingredients.
4. Bake in the preheated Air Fryer at 360 degrees F for 15 minutes. Serve right away!

284.French Toast With Blueberries And Honey

Servings: 6
Cooking Time: 20 Minutes
Ingredients:

- 1/4 cup milk
- 2 eggs
- 2 tablespoons butter, melted
- 1/2 teaspoon ground cinnamon
- 1/4 teaspoon ground cloves
- 1 teaspoon vanilla extract
- 6 slices day-old French baguette
- 2 tablespoons honey
- 1/2 cup blueberries

Directions:

1. In a mixing bowl, whisk the milk eggs, butter, cinnamon, cloves, and vanilla extract.

2. Dip each piece of the baguette into the egg mixture and place in the parchment-lined Air Fryer basket.
3. Cook in the preheated Air Fryer at 360 degrees F for 6 to 7 minutes, turning them over halfway through the cooking time to ensure even cooking.
4. Serve garnished with honey and blueberries. Enjoy!

285.Old-fashioned Beef Stroganoff

Servings: 4
Cooking Time: 20 Minutes
Ingredients:
- 3/4 pound beef sirloin steak, cut into small-sized strips
- 1/4 cup balsamic vinegar
- 1 tablespoon brown mustard
- 2 tablespoons all-purpose flour
- 1 tablespoon butter
- 1 cup beef broth
- 1 cup leek, chopped
- 2 cloves garlic, crushed
- 1 teaspoon cayenne pepper
- Sea salt flakes and crushed red pepper, to taste
- 1 cup sour cream
- 2 ½ tablespoons tomato paste

Directions:
1. Place the beef along with the balsamic vinegar and the mustard in a mixing dish; cover and marinate in your refrigerator for about 1 hour.
2. Then, coat the beef strips with the flour; butter the inside of a baking dish and put the beef into the dish.
3. Add the broth, leeks and garlic. Cook at 380 degrees for 8 minutes. Pause the machine and add the cayenne pepper, salt, red pepper, sour cream

and tomato paste; cook for additional 7 minutes.
4. Check for doneness and serve with warm egg noodles, if desired. Bon appétit!

286.Mediterranean Eggs With Spinach And Tomato

Servings: 2
Cooking Time: 15 Minutes
Ingredients:
- 2 tablespoons olive oil, melted
- 4 eggs, whisked
- 5 ounces fresh spinach, chopped
- 1 medium-sized tomato, chopped
- 1 teaspoon fresh lemon juice
- 1/2 teaspoon coarse salt
- 1/2 teaspoon ground black pepper
- 1/2 cup of fresh basil, roughly chopped

Directions:
1. Add the olive oil to an Air Fryer baking pan. Make sure to tilt the pan to spread the oil evenly.
2. Simply combine the remaining ingredients, except for the basil leaves; whisk well until everything is well incorporated.
3. Cook in the preheated Air Fryer for 8 to 12 minutes at 280 degrees F. Garnish with fresh basil leaves. Serve warm with a dollop of sour cream if desired.

287.Famous Cheese And Bacon Rolls

Servings: 6
Cooking Time: 10 Minutes
Ingredients:
- 1/3 cup Swiss cheese, shredded
- 10 slices of bacon
- 10 ounces canned crescent rolls
- 2 tablespoons yellow mustard 6

Directions:

1. Start by preheating your air fryer to 325 degrees F.
2. Then, form the crescent rolls into "sheets". Spread mustard over the sheets. Place the chopped Swiss cheese and bacon in the middle of each dough sheet.
3. Create the rolls and bake them for about 9 minutes.
4. Then, set the machine to 385 degrees F; bake for an additional 4 minutes in the preheated air fryer. Eat warm with some extra yellow mustard.

288.Cheesy Zucchini With Queso Añejo

Servings: 4
Cooking Time: 25 Minutes
Ingredients:

- 1 large-sized zucchini, thinly sliced
- 1/4 cup almond flour
- 1 cup parmesan cheese
- 1 egg, whisked
- 1/2 cup Queso Añejo, grated
- Salt and cracked pepper, to taste

Directions:

1. Pat dry the zucchini slices with a kitchen towel.
2. Mix the remaining ingredients in a shallow bowl; mix until everything is well combined. Dip each zucchini slice in the prepared batter.
3. Cook in the preheated Air Fryer at 400 degrees F for 12 minutes, shaking the basket halfway through the cooking time.
4. Work in batches until the zucchini slices are crispy and golden brown. Enjoy!

289.Cheese Sticks With Ketchup

Servings: 4

Cooking Time: 15 Minutes
Ingredients:

- 1/4 cup coconut flour
- 1/4 cup almond flour
- 2 eggs
- 1/2 cup parmesan cheese, grated
- 1 tablespoon Cajun seasonings
- 8 cheese sticks, kid-friendly
- 1/4 cup ketchup, low-carb

Directions:

1. To begin, set up your breading station. Place the flour in a shallow dish. In a separate dish, whisk the eggs.
2. Finally, mix the parmesan cheese and Cajun seasoning in a third dish.
3. Start by dredging the cheese sticks in the flour; then, dip them into the egg. Press the cheese sticks into the parmesan mixture, coating evenly.
4. Place the breaded cheese sticks in the lightly greased Air Fryer basket. Cook at 380 degrees F for 6 minutes.
5. Serve with ketchup and enjoy!

290.Baked Eggs With Kale And Ham

Servings: 2
Cooking Time: 15 Minutes
Ingredients:

- 2 eggs
- 1/4 teaspoon dried or fresh marjoram
- 2 teaspoons chili powder
- 1/3 teaspoon kosher salt
- ½ cup steamed kale
- 1/4 teaspoon dried or fresh rosemary
- 4 pork ham slices
- 1/3 teaspoon ground black pepper, or more to taste

Directions:

1. Divide the kale and ham among 2 ramekins; crack an egg into each ramekin. Sprinkle with seasonings.
2. Cook for 15 minutes at 335 degrees F or until your eggs reach desired texture.
3. Serve warm with spicy tomato ketchup and pickles. Bon appétit!

291.All-in-one Spicy Spaghetti With Beef

Servings: 4
Cooking Time: 30 Minutes
Ingredients:
- 3/4 pound ground chuck
- 1 onion, peeled and finely chopped
- 1 teaspoon garlic paste
- 1 bell pepper, chopped
- 1 small-sized habanero pepper, deveined and finely minced
- 1/2 teaspoon dried rosemary
- 1/2 teaspoon dried marjoram
- 1 ¼ cups crushed tomatoes, fresh or canned
- 1/2 teaspoon sea salt flakes
- 1/4 teaspoon ground black pepper, or more to taste
- 1 package cooked spaghetti, to serve

Directions:
1. In the Air Fryer baking dish, place the ground meat, onion, garlic paste, bell pepper, habanero pepper, rosemary, and the marjoram.
2. Air-fry, uncovered, for 10 to 11 minutes. Next step, stir in the tomatoes along with salt and pepper; cook 17 to 20 minutes. Serve over cooked spaghetti. Bon appétit!

292.Baked Denver Omelet With Sausage

Servings: 5
Cooking Time: 14 Minutes
Ingredients:
- 3 pork sausages, chopped
- 8 well-beaten eggs
- 1 ½ bell peppers, seeded and chopped
- 1 teaspoon smoked cayenne pepper
- 2 tablespoons Fontina cheese
- 1/2 teaspoon tarragon
- 1/2 teaspoon ground black pepper
- 1 teaspoon salt

Directions:
1. In a cast-iron skillet, sweat the bell peppers together with the chopped pork sausages until the peppers are fragrant and the sausage begins to release liquid.
2. Lightly grease the inside of a baking dish with pan spray.
3. Throw all of the above ingredients into the prepared baking dish, including the sautéed mixture; stir to combine.
4. Bake at 345 degrees F approximately 9 minutes. Serve right away with the salad of choice.

293.Fingerling Potatoes With Cashew Sauce

Servings: 4
Cooking Time: 20 Minutes
Ingredients:
- 1 pound fingerling potatoes
- 1 tablespoon butter, melted
- Sea salt and ground black pepper, to your liking
- 1 teaspoon shallot powder
- 1 teaspoon garlic powder
- Cashew Sauce:
- 1/2 cup raw cashews
- 1 teaspoon cayenne pepper
- 3 tablespoons nutritional yeast
- 2 teaspoons white vinegar

- 4 tablespoons water
- 1/4 teaspoon dried rosemary
- 1/4 teaspoon dried dill

Directions:
1. Toss the potatoes with the butter, salt, black pepper, shallot powder, and garlic powder.
2. Place the fingerling potatoes in the lightly greased Air Fryer basket and cook at 400 degrees F for 6 minutes; shake the basket and cook for a further 6 minutes.
3. Meanwhile, make the sauce by mixing all ingredients in your food processor or high-speed blender.
4. Drizzle the cashew sauce over the potato wedges. Bake at 400 degrees F for 2 more minutes or until everything is heated through. Enjoy!

294. Muffins With Brown Mushrooms

Servings: 6
Cooking Time: 25 Minutes
Ingredients:
- 2 tablespoons butter, melted
- 1 yellow onion, chopped
- 2 garlic cloves, minced
- 1 cup brown mushrooms, sliced
- Sea salt and ground black pepper, to taste
- 1 teaspoon fresh basil
- 8 eggs, lightly whisked
- 6 ounces goat cheese, crumbled

Directions:
1. Start by preheating your Air Fryer to 330 degrees F. Now, spritz a 6-tin muffin tin with cooking spray.
2. Melt the butter in a heavy-bottomed skillet over medium-high heat. Sauté the onions, garlic, and mushrooms until just tender and fragrant.

3. Add the salt, black pepper, and basil and remove from heat. Divide out the sautéed mixture into the muffin tin.
4. Pour the whisked eggs on top and top with the goat cheese. Bake for 20 minutes rotating the pan halfway through the cooking time. Bon appétit!

295. Traditional Onion Bhaji

Servings: 3
Cooking Time: 40 Minutes
Ingredients:
- 1 egg, beaten
- 2 tablespoons olive oil
- 2 onions, sliced
- 1 green chili, deseeded and finely chopped
- 2 ounces chickpea flour
- 1 ounce all-purpose flour
- Salt and black pepper, to taste
- 1 teaspoon cumin seeds
- 1/2 teaspoon ground turmeric

Directions:
1. Place all ingredients, except for the onions, in a mixing dish; mix to combine well, adding a little water to the mixture.
2. Once you've got a thick batter, add the onions; stir to coat well.
3. Cook in the preheated Air Fryer at 370 degrees F for 20 minutes flipping them halfway through the cooking time.
4. Work in batches and transfer to a serving platter. Enjoy!

296. Grilled Lemony Pork Chops

Servings: 5
Cooking Time: 34 Minutes
Ingredients:
- 5 pork chops
- 1/3 cup vermouth

- 1/2 teaspoon paprika
- 2 sprigs thyme, only leaves, crushed
- 1/2 teaspoon dried oregano
- Fresh parsley, to serve
- 1 teaspoon garlic salt½ lemon, cut into wedges
- 1 teaspoon freshly cracked black pepper
- 3 tablespoons lemon juice
- 3 cloves garlic, minced
- 2 tablespoons canola oil

Directions:
1. Firstly, heat the canola oil in a sauté pan over a moderate heat. Now, sweat the garlic until just fragrant.
2. Remove the pan from the heat and pour in the lemon juice and vermouth. Now, throw in the seasonings. Dump the sauce into a baking dish, along with the pork chops.
3. Tuck the lemon wedges among the pork chops and air-fry for 27 minutes at 345 degrees F. Bon appétit!

297.Onion Rings Wrapped In Bacon

Servings: 4
Cooking Time: 25 Minutes
Ingredients:
- 12 rashers back bacon
- 1/2 teaspoon ground black pepper
- Chopped fresh parsley, to taste
- 1/2 teaspoon paprika
- 1/2 teaspoon chili powder
- 1/2 tablespoon soy sauce
- ½ teaspoon salt

Directions:
1. Start by preheating your air fryer to 355 degrees F.
2. Season the onion rings with paprika, salt, black pepper, and chili powder.

Simply wrap the bacon around the onion rings; drizzle with soy sauce.
3. Bake for 17 minutes, garnish with fresh parsley and serve. Bon appétit!

298.Cheese Balls With Spinach

Servings: 4
Cooking Time: 15 Minutes
Ingredients:
- 1/4 cup milk
- 2 eggs
- 1 cup cheese
- 2 cups spinach, torn into pieces
- 1/3 cup flaxseed meal
- 1/2 teaspoon baking powder
- 2 tablespoons canola oil
- Salt and ground black pepper, to taste

Directions:
1. Add all the ingredients to a food processor or blender; then, puree the ingredients until it becomes dough.
2. Next, roll the dough into small balls. Preheat your air fryer to 310 degrees F.
3. Cook the balls in your Air Fryer for about 12 minutes or until they are crispy. Bon appétit!

299.Family Favorite Stuffed Mushrooms

Servings: 2
Cooking Time: 16 Minutes
Ingredients:
- 2 teaspoons cumin powder
- 4 garlic cloves, peeled and minced
- 1 small onion, peeled and chopped
- 2 tablespoons bran cereal, crushed
- 18 medium-sized white mushrooms
- Fine sea salt and freshly ground black pepper, to your liking
- A pinch ground allspice
- 2 tablespoons olive oil

Directions:

1. First, clean the mushrooms; remove the middle stalks from the mushrooms to prepare the "shells".
2. Grab a mixing dish and thoroughly combine the remaining items. Fill the mushrooms with the prepared mixture.
3. Cook the mushrooms at 345 degrees F heat for 12 minutes. Enjoy!

300.Dinner Avocado Chicken Sliders

Servings: 4
Cooking Time: 10 Minutes
Ingredients:

- ½ pounds ground chicken meat
- 4 burger buns
- 1/2 cup Romaine lettuce, loosely packed
- ½ teaspoon dried parsley flakes
- 1/3 teaspoon mustard seeds
- 1 teaspoon onion powder
- 1 ripe fresh avocado, mashed
- 1 teaspoon garlic powder
- 1 ½ tablespoon extra-virgin olive oil
- 1 cloves garlic, minced
- Nonstick cooking spray
- Salt and cracked black pepper (peppercorns, to taste

Directions:

1. Firstly, spritz an air fryer cooking basket with a nonstick cooking spray.
2. Mix ground chicken meat, mustard seeds, garlic powder, onion powder, parsley, salt, and black pepper until everything is thoroughly combined. Make sure not to overwork the meat to avoid tough chicken burgers.
3. Shape the meat mixture into patties and roll them in breadcrumbs; transfer your burgers to the prepared cooking basket. Brush the patties with the cooking spray.
4. Air-fry at 355 F for 9 minutes, working in batches. Slice burger buns into halves. In the meantime, combine olive oil with mashed avocado and pressed garlic.
5. To finish, lay Romaine lettuce and avocado spread on bun bottoms; now, add burgers and bun tops. Bon appétit!

Lightning Source UK Ltd.
Milton Keynes UK
UKHW032057241122
412811UK00008B/172